Sex tips for girls by guys

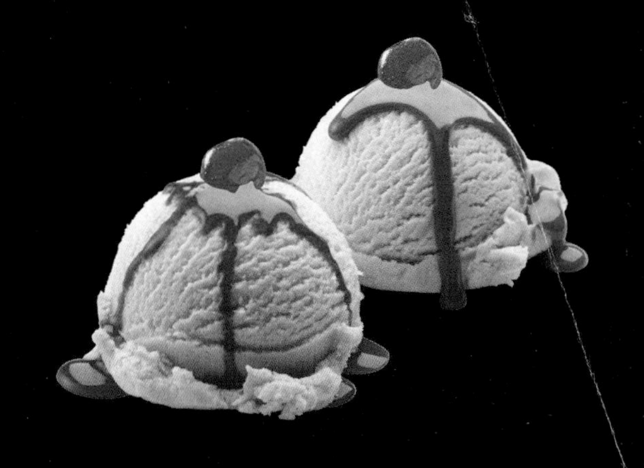

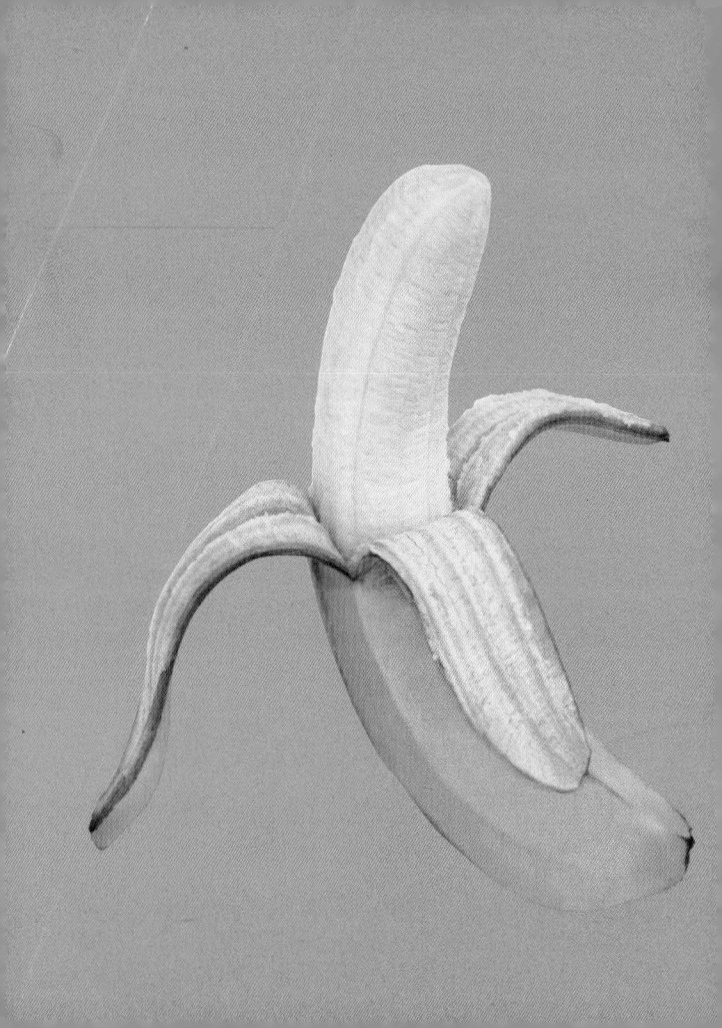

Sex tips for girls by guys

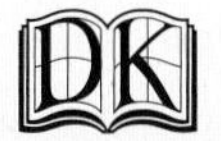

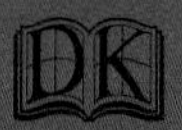

LONDON, NEW YORK, MUNICH,
MELBOURNE, DELHI

Project Editor Laura Palosuo
Editor Becky Alexander
US Editor Rachel Bozek
Project Art Editor Wendy Bartlet
Designer Nigel Wright
Managing Editor Penny Smith
Managing Art Editor Marianne Markham
Production Editor Clare McLean
Senior Production Controller Seyhan Esen
Creative Technical Support Sonia Charbonnier
Publisher Peggy Vance

This edition first published in 2012 by DK Publishing
375 Hudson Street, New York, New York 10014

12 13 14 15 16 10 9 8 7 6 5 4 3 2 1
001—182625—Jan/2012

Published in Great Britain by Dorling Kindersley Limited.

A catalog record for this book is available from the Library of Congress.
ISBN 978-0-7566-8967-4

Color reproduction by Media Development & Printing Ltd.
Printed and bound in Singapore by Tien Wah Press

contents

intro

OK, we'll let you in on a secret. It's easy to make a **guy happy** in bed. Often, just the fact that you're **pleased to be in bed** is enough to put **joy in our hearts.** So imagine what it's like when you want to **indulge us** with the tips and treats in this book. **Pure heaven.**

duction

Whether you use this book to **dip into at random** or you work through every single tip **(hint: we'd like that),** expect to have a very **happy and contented** man on your hands.

Now, isn't it time for bed...?

tou

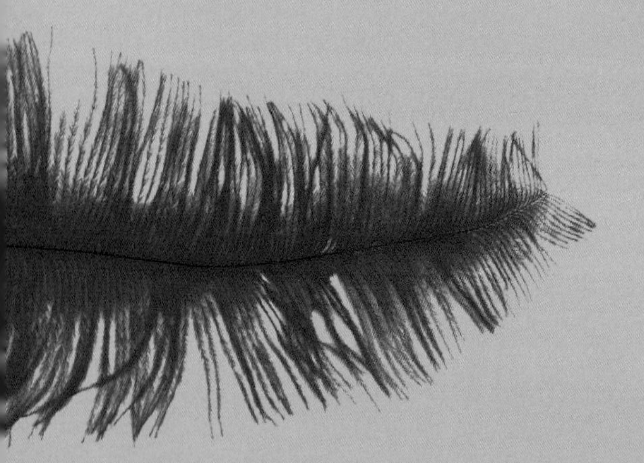

ch
me

sweet &

Like you, we love a bit of sexy foreplay before we get down to serious business.

"She came to bed **wearing just a feather boa.** She u

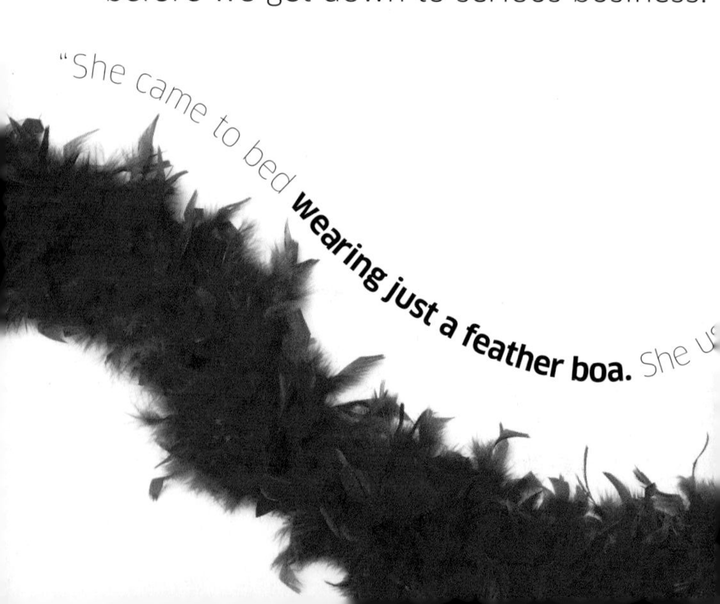

sensual

caress every part of my body. I still think about it."

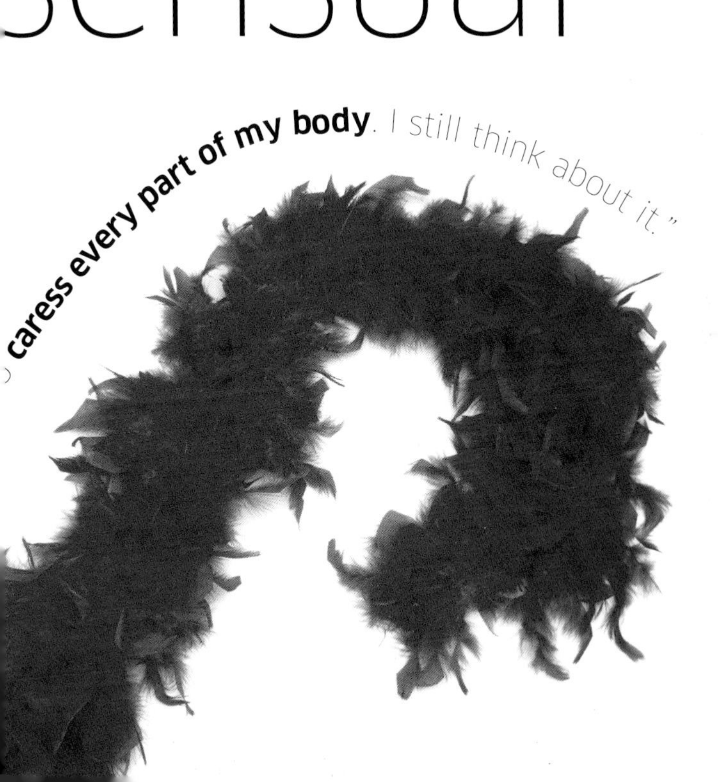

man pa

We don't often **pamper** our **bodies** so whe

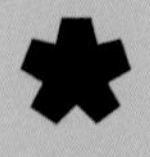

Take a **bath together.** Sit behind and **massage his back** and **chest** with **bubbles** or shower gel.

mpering

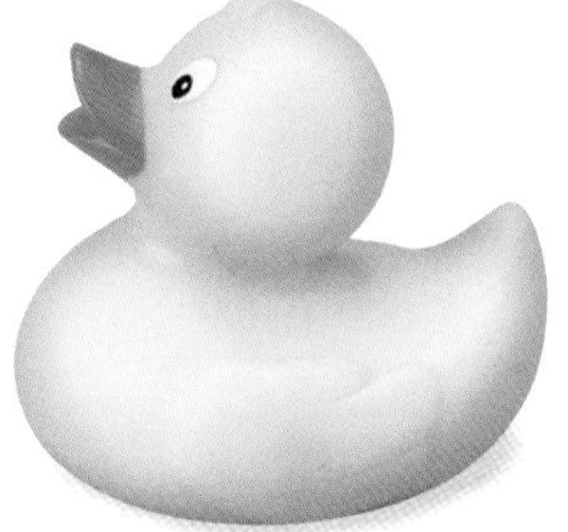

ou do it for us it feels like a **very special treat.**

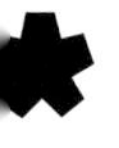

Rub massage oil **all over** him. Use firm, **confident strokes,** then try some light, **teasing strokes.**

mmmmm

You already know the headline erogenous zones. But don't forget to show some attention to our less famous parts—the ones that make us go "mmmm" with quiet satisfaction.

✱ **"She kisses me** on my jawline and then slowly **works her way down** the side of my neck. **It feels amazing."**

zones

✱ "She moves her **fingertip over my lips,** then **gently pushes** her finger **into my mouth."**

✱ "She **rakes my pubes** with her **fingernails**, nearly **touching my penis,** but not quite."

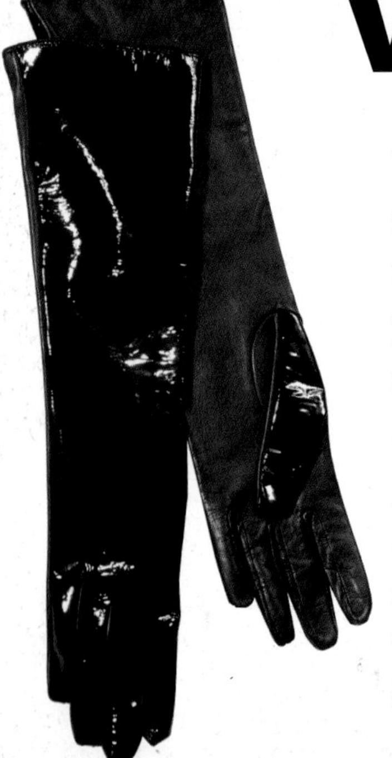

very

Taking us in hand is a skill we'll love you for. It's thrilling to feel your touch. And that means casual strokes as well as full-on hand jobs. Stroke, caress, and squeeze us with soft, bare hands—or wear sexy gloves for a different touch.

handy

✱ **Say hello** by sneaking your **hands around his waist** from behind. Trace the **outline of his package** while pressing **your breasts** against his back. Now **slip your fingers** into **his pants** and tease him with a **few light strokes.**

✱ **Join him** for a **shower,** squirt some shower gel into **your palms,** and **massage his penis** using long strokes.

two

We like it when you mix things up a bit. Even something simple like using two hands rather than one makes us sit up and take notice.

handers

✱ "She puts **massage oil in her hands** and wraps both hands **around my erection**. Then she **twists gently** in opposite directions. **Feels fantastic."**

✱ **"She does this great move** where she links her fingers together and then her hands **glide up and down."**

✱ "She sits **between my legs** and **strokes my penis** hand over hand. **So sexy!"**

f

There's one particular part of the penis–the F-spot–that really gets our attention. It's that place on the underside where the foreskin joins the penis, aka the "banjo string."

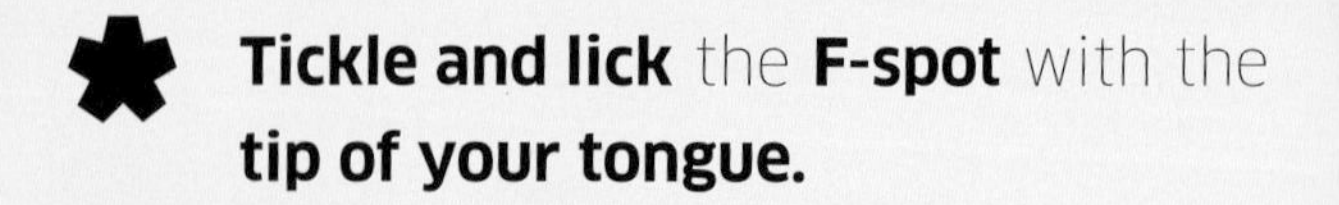

✱ **Tickle and lick** the **F-spot** with the **tip of your tongue.**

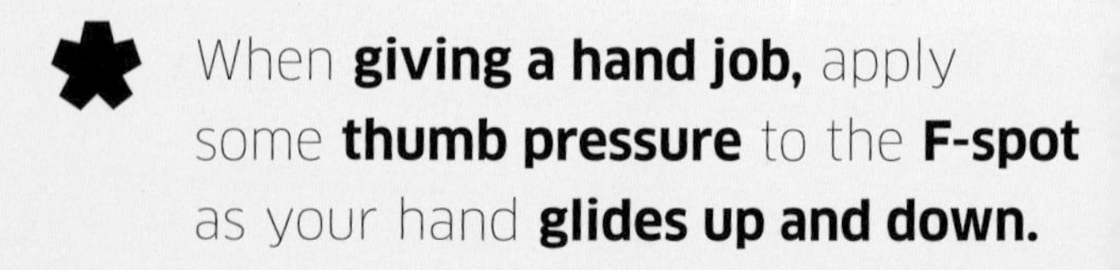

✱ When **giving a hand job,** apply some **thumb pressure** to the **F-spot** as your hand **glides up and down.**

spotting

✱ Lick your **index finger,** then draw **tiny, wet circles** on his **F-spot.**

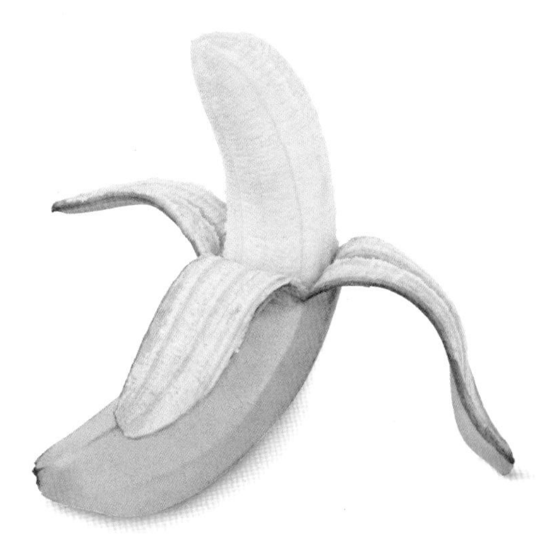

happy

As much as we love a bit of hand-to-penis attention during foreplay, we sometimes like a hand job to go all the way. Lying back and looking forward to a happy ending can be sheer bliss.

"There's **something thrilling** about the way she literally **takes me in hand** and **takes control."**

endings

"When I'm in the **home stretch,** I like **hard, fast pumps** around the head that don't **change in speed."**

"It's a cliché, but it drives me wild to **come on her breasts."**

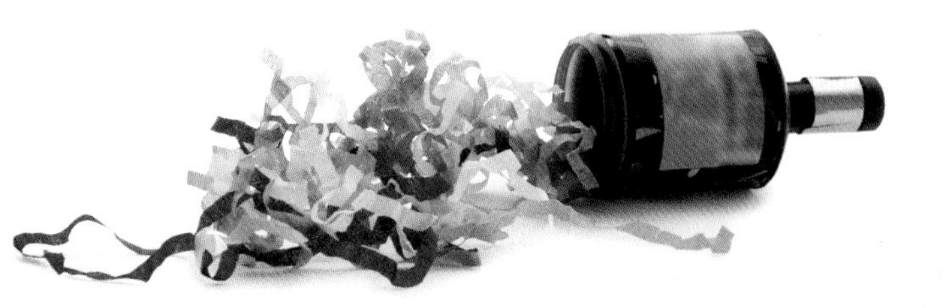

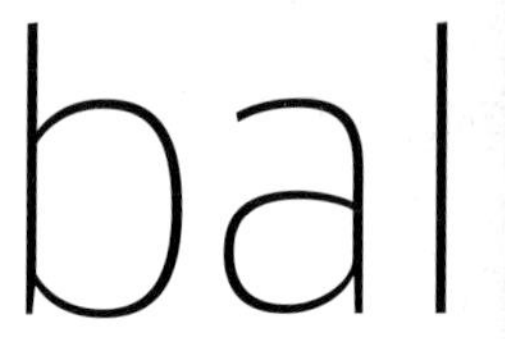

Our balls are very close to the dance floor but they don't always get invited to the party, which is a shame. They're packed with nerve endings and we love it when you play with them.

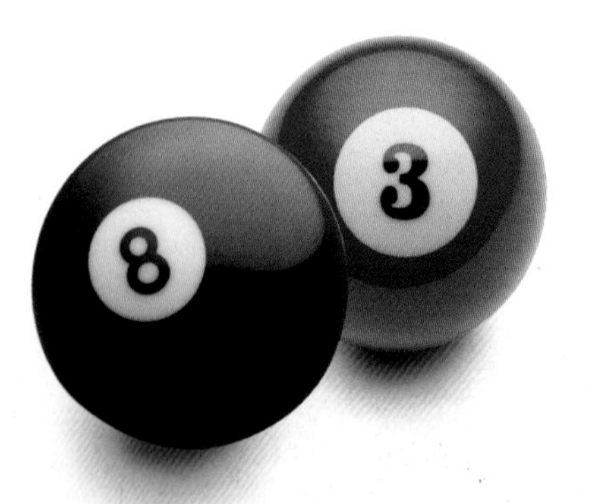

play

✱ Try **treating the boys** to any or all of these: **barely-there cat licks; sucks** and **kisses;** light grazing with **your fingernails;** or a nice **snug hold** in the **palm of your hand.**

✱ We're also fans of **sex positions** that are **ball-inclusive.** Try sitting **on top** and **sliding back and forth.** Also, when you stand up and bend over, **our crown jewels give a gentle slap** with each inward thrust.

no-man's

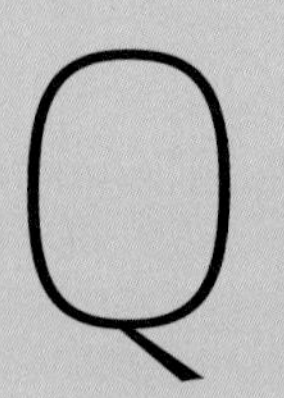

Name one part of a man that rarely gets touched.

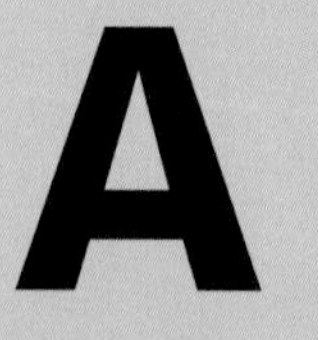

The stretch of skin behind his balls. Men call it the "taint" because "it ain't balls and it ain't ass."

land

* Make it **your mission** to discover this lost erogenous zone: **Caress his taint** with **your fingers** or **tongue.**

* **The taint** is also an **excellent resting spot** when you want to calm him down **during a blow job.** Treat him to **some soft kisses** down there before you return to the main action.

We love it when you do a little exploring down under. Let your fingers trail down the penis, over the balls, and do a little teasing of the anus.

under

Stroke or **circle his anus** with a lightly **lubed finger.** Experiment with applying a **little more pressure** or venturing a **short way inside.**

Always pay attention to **his body language** and let it be your guide. Tightly **clenched buttocks** means **"no thanks"** while **lifting his pelvis** toward you says **"go right ahead."**

umop

inside **job**

Know your G-spot? Well, we've got one, too. It's called the P-spot and, if you know where to find it, you can unlock a mind-blowing orgasm.

Gently insert your finger into **his anus.** **Reach up and forward** (toward his belly). Let his **moans of pleasure** guide you to the **right spot.** While you're busy in the basement, get him to **pleasure himself** up top. Or give him a **blow job.** Either way, the results will be **bed-rocking.**

getting

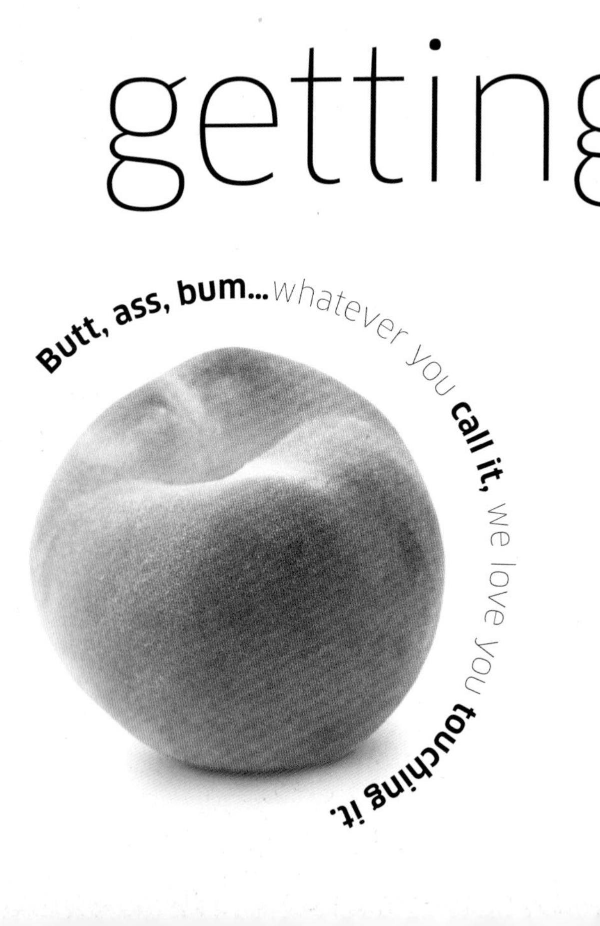

cheeky

✱ Give him a **bare-butt massage.** Use your palms to **press**, **pound**, **and pummel**, and then change the pace by **tracing your fingertips** lightly across his skin for a **sexy contrast.**

✱ **Try hands-free:** Rub massage oil over **your belly and breasts** and then slither up and down on his back and backside. **Warning: He may roll over and grab you...**

master class

If you're unsure of how a man really wants to be handled, there's a simple way to find out: Ask for a demo. Chances are he will be very willing to oblige.

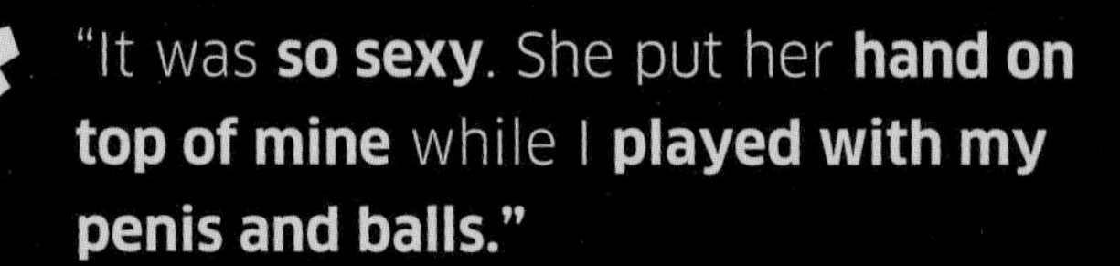

"It was **so sexy**. She put her **hand on top of mine** while I **played with my penis and balls."**

"She laid **in between my legs** and asked to **watch me masturbate.** I loved it! It's usually **me who tries to watch!"**

nipple

Our nipples may not be quite as sensitive as yours, but they're still a hot spot. Like you, we get more of a sensation if you prepare the ground. So here are some nipple play tips!

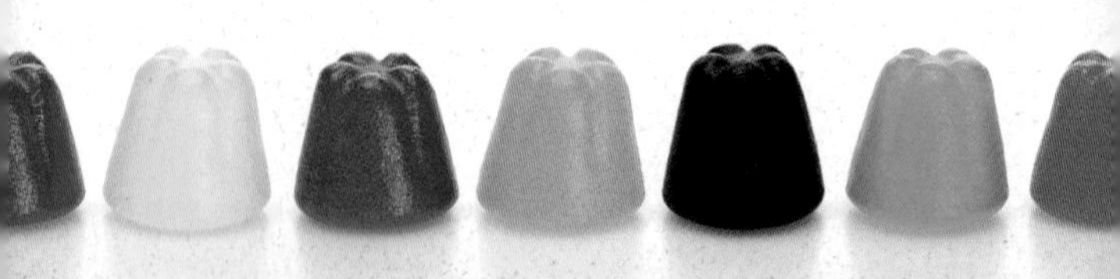

play

We **like it** when you **mix up the sensations.** Start by **licking,** then try **nibbling.** Or **stroke gently** with your fingertips, followed by a **pinch.**

Try **licking a nipple**, then **blowing** across it to give us the **good kind of goosebumps.**

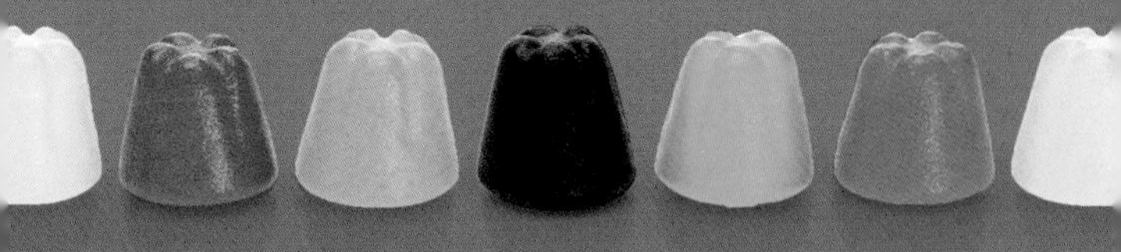

heady sens

Not that kind of head. The scalp. A head massage will relax us and leave us like putty in your hands.

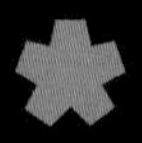

Sit on the floor with **his head** in your lap. **Glide your fingertips** firmly along his hairline. Now **circle his temples.** Repeat until **he purrs.**

ations

✱ Do this in your **underwear** or **naked** for an **extra wow factor.**

✱ **Finish your massage** by leaning forward to deliver **a passionate kiss.**

✱ Try giving a **head massage** when we are **facedown** in **your lap.**

toe play

Despite its dubious reputation, toe play can make grown men groan. Why? Because it reminds us of a blow job. So ramp up the associations with lots of licking and sucking.

Give us **a sexy look** while you do **some mouth-toe play.** Add some playful licks, and let your **lips slide up and down** with **titillating slowness.**

A shared bath (or hot tub) is a great venue **for toe sucking**. Sit at opposite ends and **take his foot firmly** in hand. (You can wash his feet first then, too...)

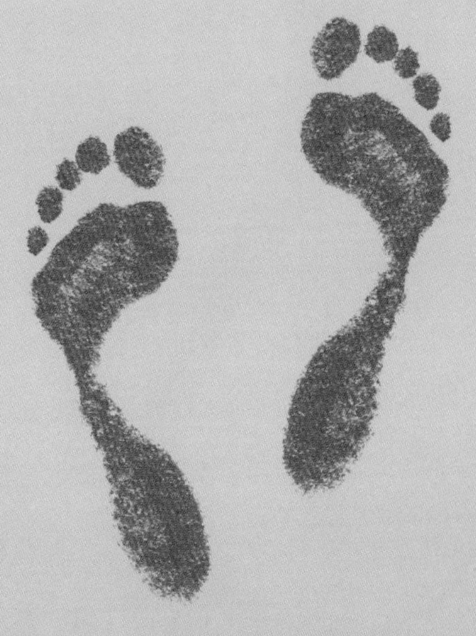

no

If you've **got long hair,** let it trail **over his chest.**

handers

Who says a massage has to be done with hands alone? Feel free to rub other parts of your body against us, too.

* Try **getting on all fours** above him and **caressing him** with your **breasts.** The **soft, stroking** sensations will **drive him to distraction.**

* **Play footsie.** Your feet can deliver amazing sensations, too—try using your toes to **lightly caress his penis.**

rough &

Sometimes we like it playful: A bit of rough-and-tumble turns us on. And we really like it when you're the boss.

- Push him **onto the bed** and pin his **arms above his head**. Move in for a **killer kiss.**

- **Flip him** onto his front and give him a **firm spank** on his **butt cheeks.** Ask innocently, **"Oh, did that hurt?"**

ready

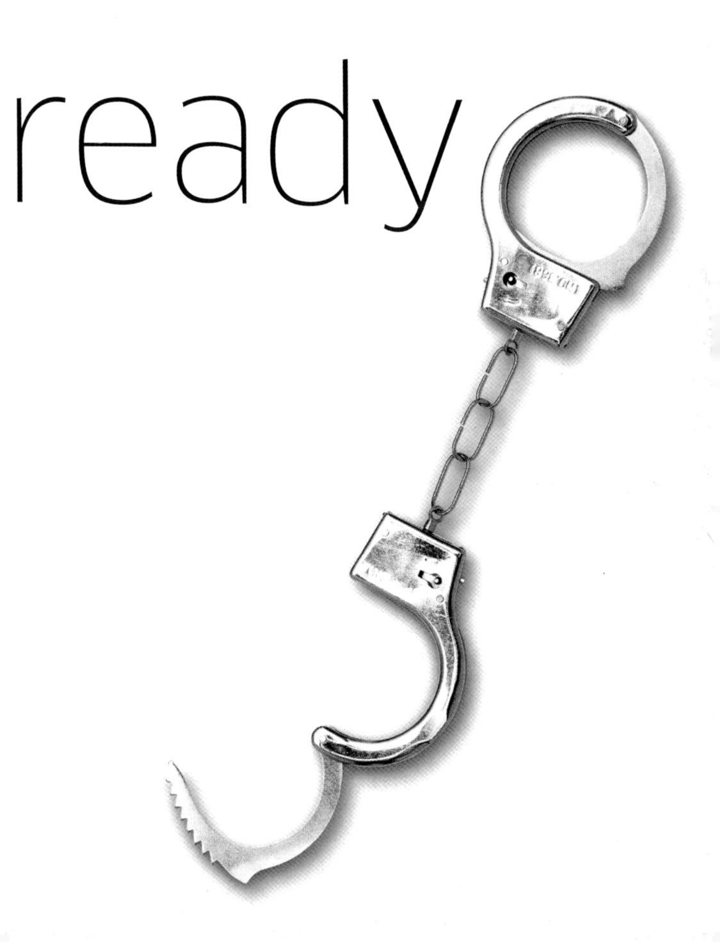

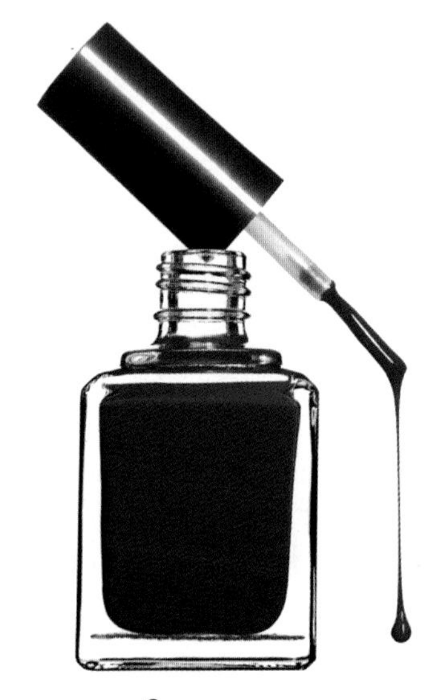

getting

What do girls have that guys don't? Long fingernails, of course. They can deliver some sexy sensations.

✱ **"She straddles me** when I'm on my front and **lightly grazes my back** with **her nails.** Makes me **shiver."**

✱ "We were getting **pretty rough** and **playful**—I woke up the **next morning** with **scratches** all over **my chest.** A hot reminder of the night before!"

scratchy

triple

If you want to make him cross-eyed with pleasure, try this advanced massage trick.

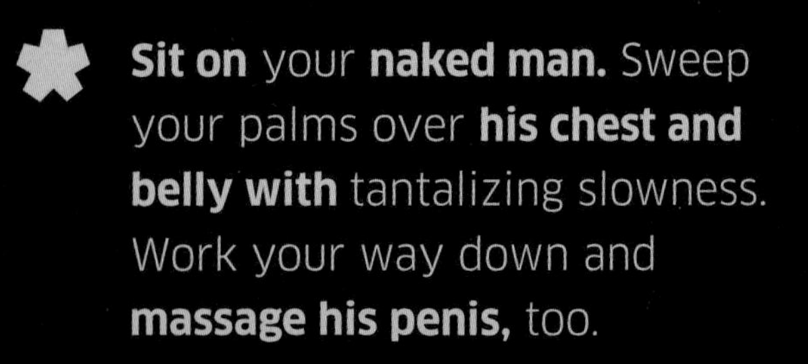

Sit on your **naked man.** Sweep your palms over **his chest and belly with** tantalizing slowness. Work your way down and **massage his penis,** too.

treat

✱ When **his flagpole** is firmly **raised, climb on board.** Continue **stroking his chest** with your palms.

✱ Move **up and down** in sync with your hands as they **travel over his body. That** is a **thorough massage.**

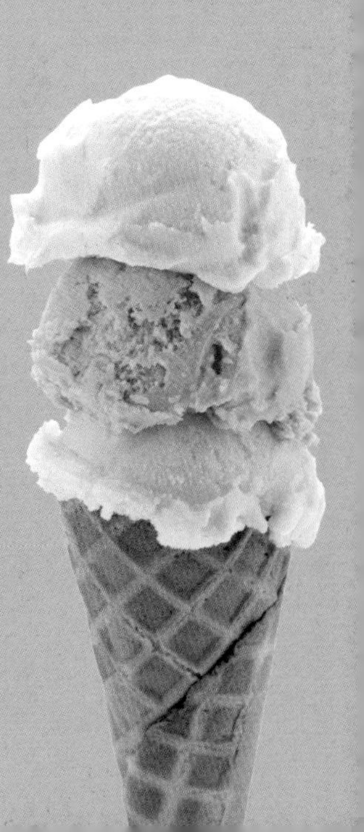

tea

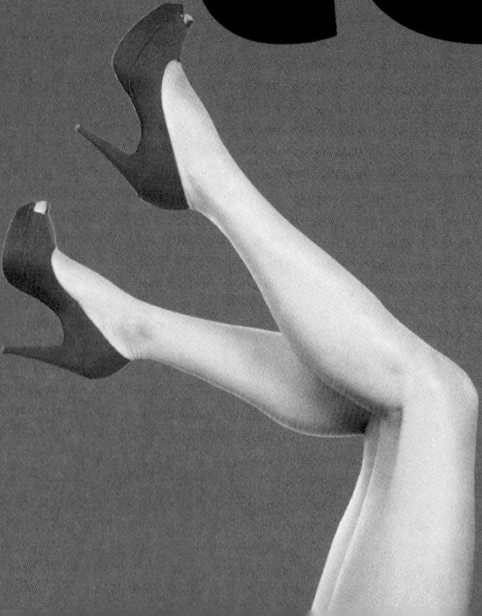

se
me

tongue

Your tongue is one of your sexiest assets. It's warm and wet and we love everything it can do. Kissing, blow jobs, neck nuzzling, toe sucking...yes, we are big fans.

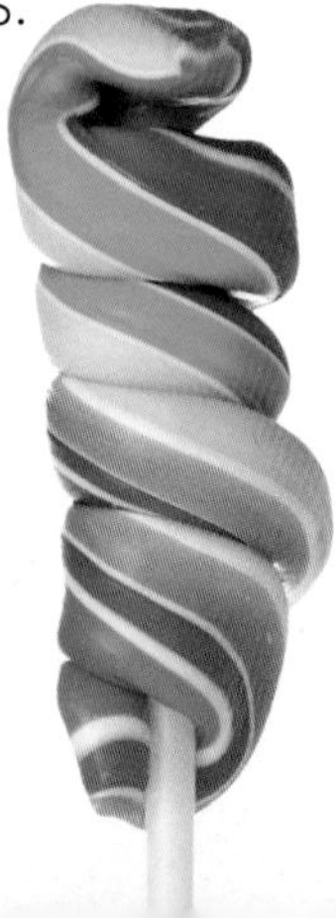

teasing

* “We were **lying on the sofa** watching TV and she raised **my hand** to **her mouth**. She **sucked each of my fingers**, one by one. **Amazing.”**

* “She **nibbled my earlobe** and I felt **her tongue** darting in my ear. Then she **took me to bed**—fantastic.”

* “She makes me **lie on my front**—then she **bites, licks,** and **nibbles** her way down my body. **Best massage ever.”**

it's in

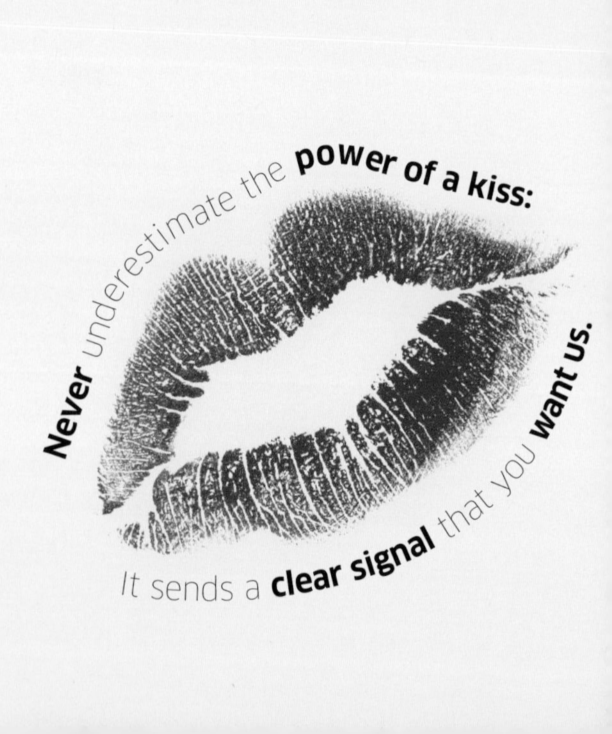
Never underestimate the **power of a kiss:**
It sends a **clear signal** that you **want us.**

her kiss

* Cup his face **sweetly** in **your hands**, give him your best **smoldering look**, and **kiss gently.** Feel your way **into his mouth** with your **tongue.** Make your **kiss long** and **sensual**—if he pulls away, **tell him "more..."**.

* **Ramp things up** by pushing him **against the nearest wall** and giving him a **sexy smooch.** Press your **pelvis hard against his** for a guaranteed **erection-starter.**

tongue slap

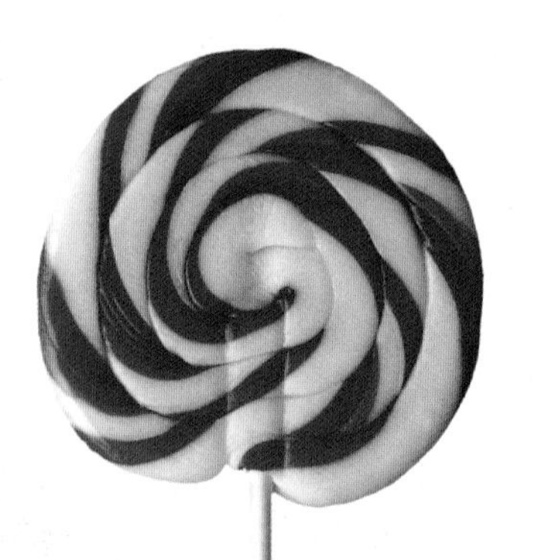

This has a slightly kinky feel to it, which is probably why we like it so much. All you need is a sexy attitude, a wet tongue, and a naked man.

Grasp his penis and stick **your tongue** out as far as you can. Give him a **wicked look.** Now **slap the head of his penis** against the **flat of your tongue.** Repeat a few times, but not too fast—you want to build up lots of **sexy anticipation** between each slap. Visually, this **looks amazingly dirty.** Plus the **wet slap** feels **fantastic.**

U-spott

Our U-spot (the eye of the penis) may be small, but it can bring us a lot of joy, so please give it a little attention.

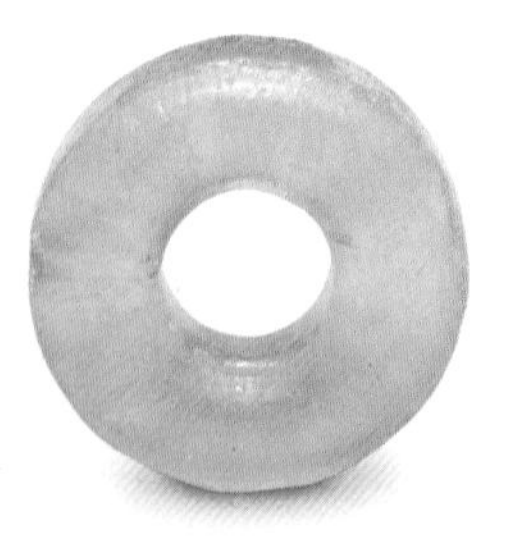

ng

✱ We **like it** when you give the U-spot some **special attention** at the **start of a blow job**; we are still **nice and sensitive** then, so can feel everything.

✱ Position the **tip of your tongue** right above the **head of the penis.** Hover for a few seconds, then draw **tiny circles around the U-spot** with the tip of your tongue. (Look up and add a **nasty wink** if you like.)

cool se

When things are getting hot and feverish, cooling things down can send a bolt of pleasure through us.

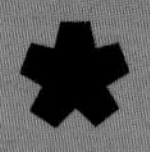

During a **back massage,** run your warm, **wet tongue** down **his spine.** Then blow cool air along the same path. Other superb **spots for licking and blowing** are his **neck and nipples.**

nsations

To **spice up a blow job,** pull away and blow a long, **cool stream of air** over **his manhood.** His hot **skin will tingle** in a way that **makes him gasp.**

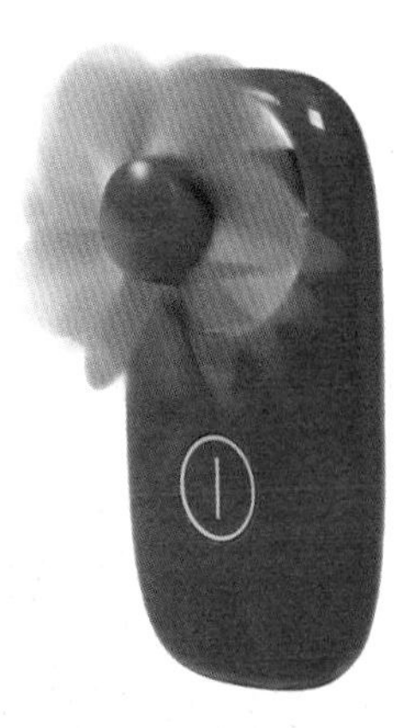

the first rule of blow jobs

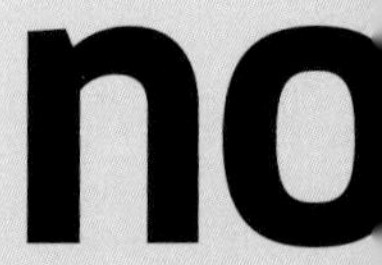

Except **gentle nibbling** by prior arrangement.

teeth

a trip **down south**

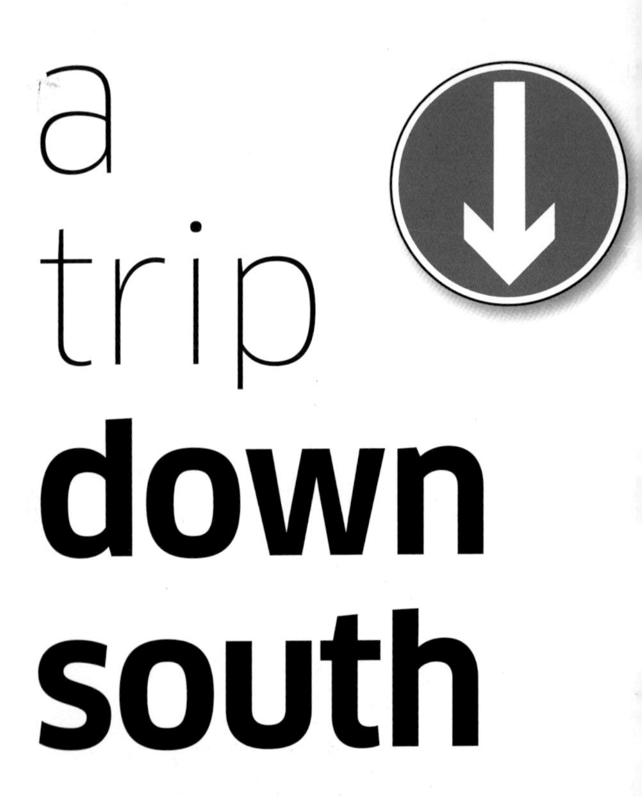

Sometimes it's about the journey and not just the destination. As your gorgeous lips travel down south, we love to be teased and tantalized on the way.

- "She makes it seem like **she's going down on me,** but then she keeps heading **back up for a kiss.** It drives me **crazy with lust."**

- "She **crawled slowly** over my body **on all fours**—her head facing my feet. She told me, 'Look but don't touch.'"

- "She kissed my toes, then worked her way up the **inside of my leg.** I could feel her **hot breath on my penis."**

quick

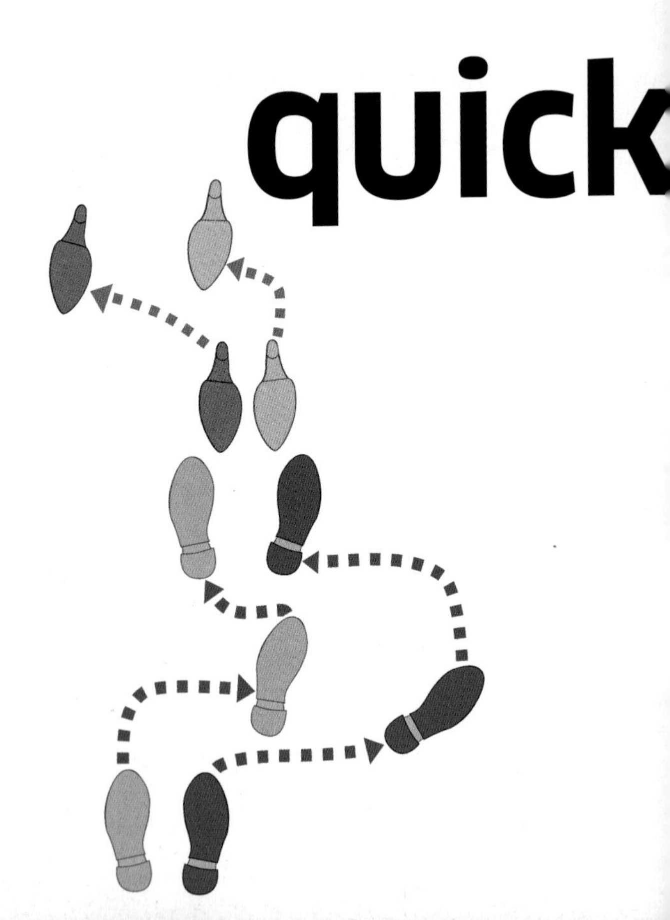

quick slow

his is all about surprise and anticipation. nd it sure beats ballroom dancing.

Do **nine quick shallow thrusts** during a **blow job,** then on your tenth stroke, **plunge your lips** as far down **his shaft** as you can. Keep everything **hot, wet, and slick,** and see him **lose control.**

swallow

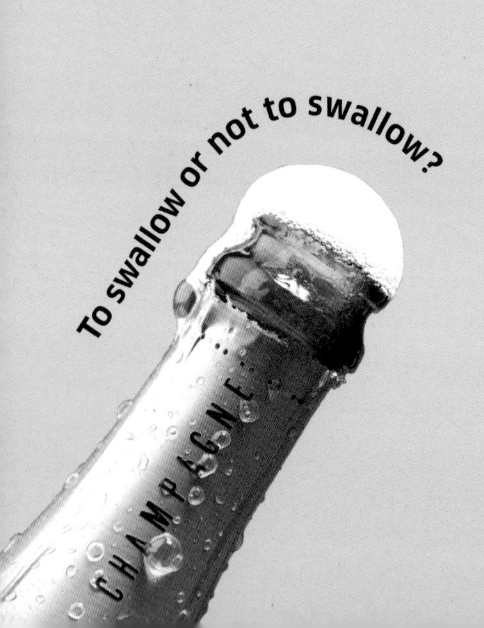

ng up

Some men are **hooked** on the idea of you **drinking their nectar.** Others are just glad you're **down there.** Ask him what he likes but most will also be happy with this:

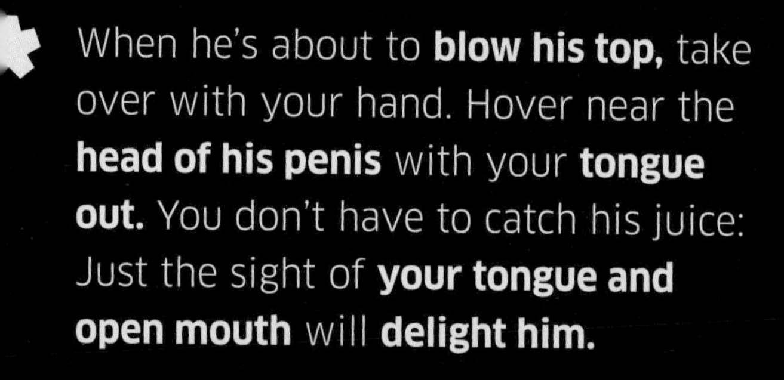

✽ When he's about to **blow his top,** take over with your hand. Hover near the **head of his penis** with your **tongue out.** You don't have to catch his juice: Just the sight of **your tongue and open mouth** will **delight him.**

Want to give him a different blow job experience? It's simple: Stay still and let him make the moves. He'll love the sensation of having some say in things.

motion

Get him to **stand up** while you **kneel in front** of him. Take **his penis** in your **mouth.** Grip with **your lips,** and keep your head still.

control

He gets to move back and forth but you stay in control. Use **your hands** to influence the **pace, depth, and rhythm.**

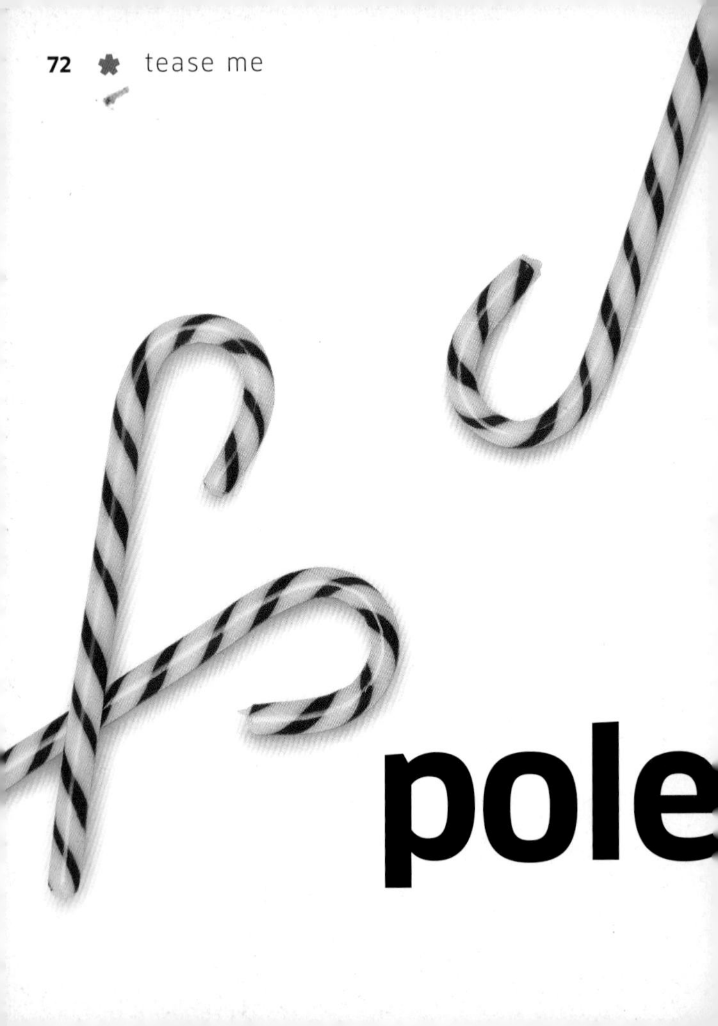

pole

We love any BJ, but if you want a new position, we're big fans of these, too:

- **"I sit** on the edge of my **office chair,** then **she kneels** on the floor **between my legs** and unzips me..."

- "I get **on all fours** on the bed and she slides in **underneath me."**

position

back of

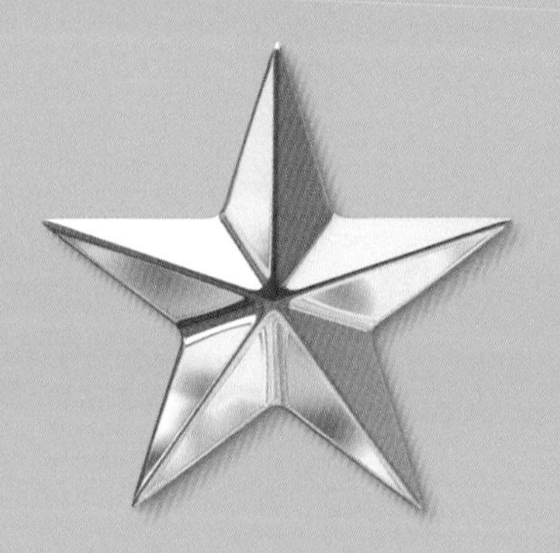

It's not everyone's idea of fun, but for paid-up members of the analingus club, nothing compares to the bliss of being licked in this oh-so-private place.

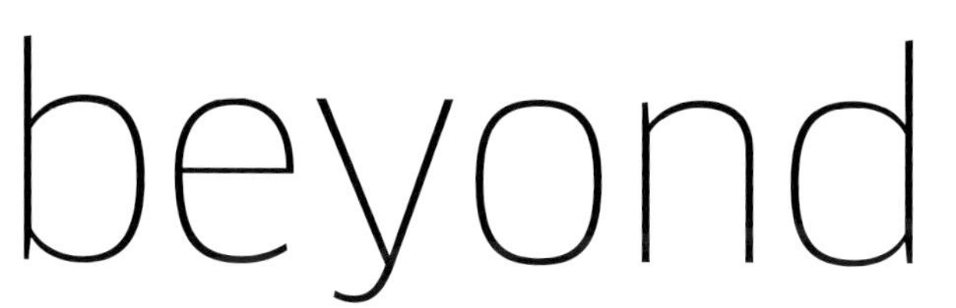

beyond

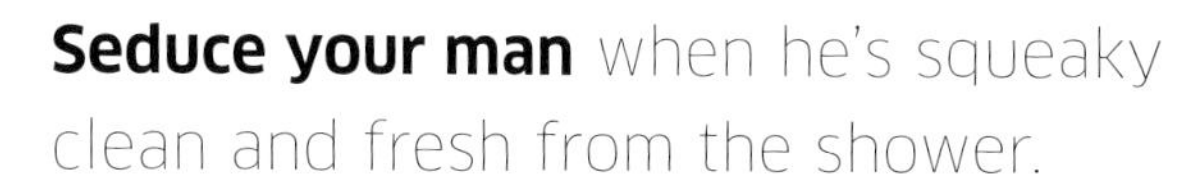

Seduce your man when he's squeaky clean and fresh from the shower. **Take your tongue** on a **sexy detour** from his **penis to his perineum**. Flick your tongue across **his star.**

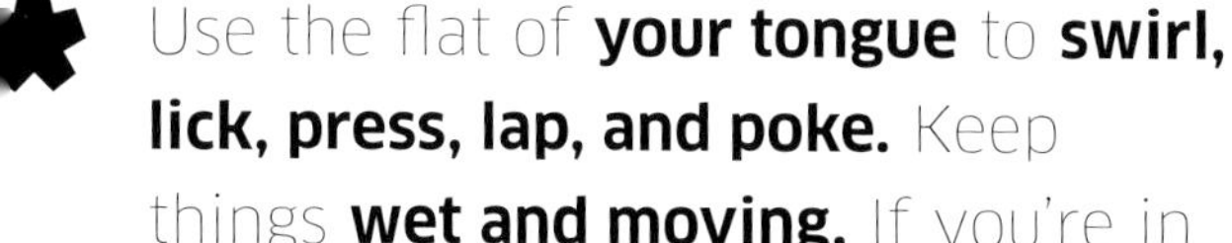

Use the flat of **your tongue** to **swirl, lick, press, lap, and poke.** Keep things **wet and moving.** If you're in the right position, lend a hand for some **top deck stimulation,** too.

glorious

Don't be shy of inviting us for a 69—we love all that mutual licking. In fact, don't even ask: Just position your body in a way that makes 69 an option we can't resist.

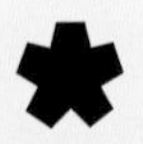

For a **chilled-out option**, lie **top-to-tail** on your sides. Get comfy with your **heads** resting on **each other's thighs,** then try some **licking.**

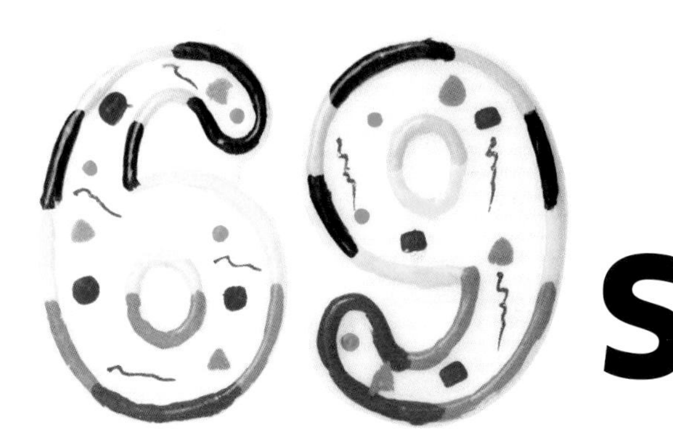

s

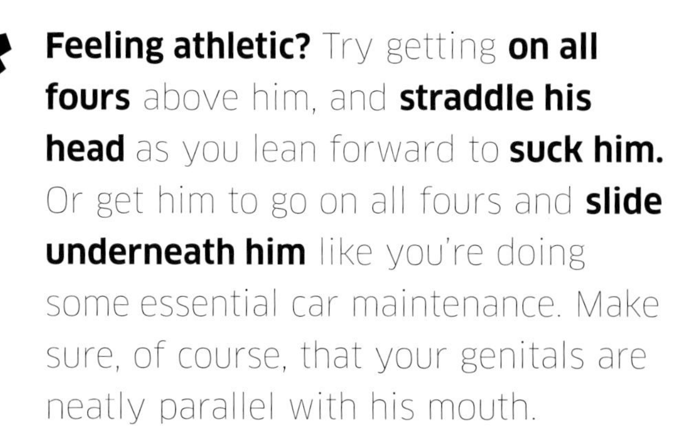

Feeling athletic? Try getting **on all fours** above him, and **straddle his head** as you lean forward to **suck him.** Or get him to go on all fours and **slide underneath him** like you're doing some essential car maintenance. Make sure, of course, that your genitals are neatly parallel with his mouth.

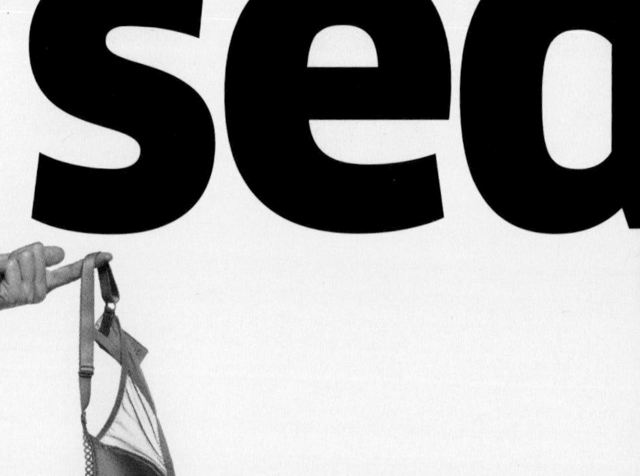
sed

uce

me

play

It's a cliché, but it's true: You want what you can't have. Even just a hint of "will she? won't she?" will send our lust levels soaring.

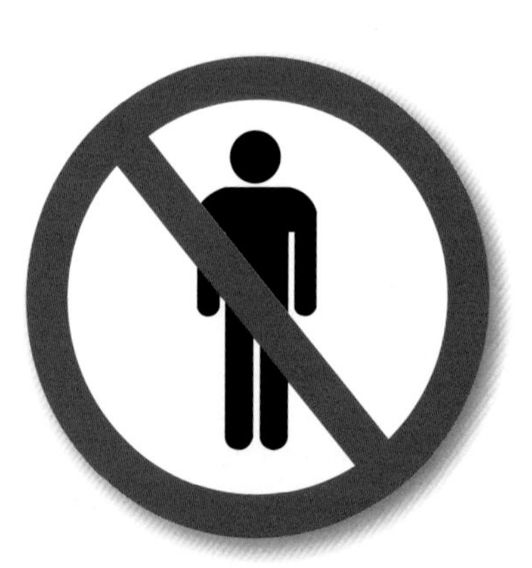

hard **to get**

"My **girlfriend** goes around the house wearing **sexy lingerie.** I try to get her into bed, but she just says, **'No chance!'** It **makes me wildly horny."**

"I asked her to come to bed, and she **smiled and refused** until I'd told her exactly how I would **pleasure her."**

top

Guys love to see sexy confidence in a girl. It shows us that you're at home in your body and you think sex is fun.

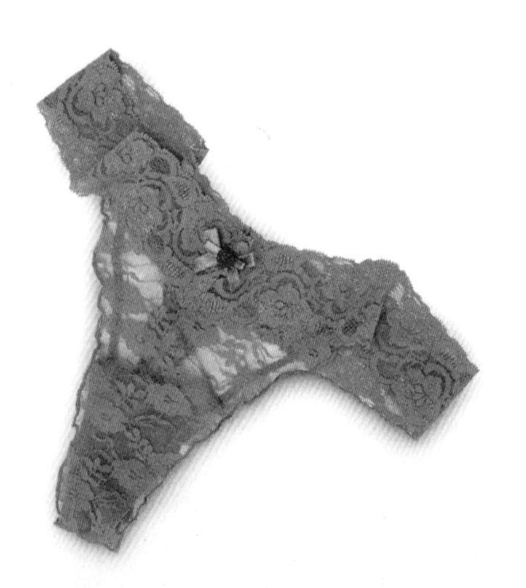

turn-ons

- If you **want him really badly,** tell him **exactly** that. **Your compliment** will go **straight** to **his genitals.**

- **Undress slooowly.** Give him a chance to **feast his eyes** on your body. And **enjoy** being watched.

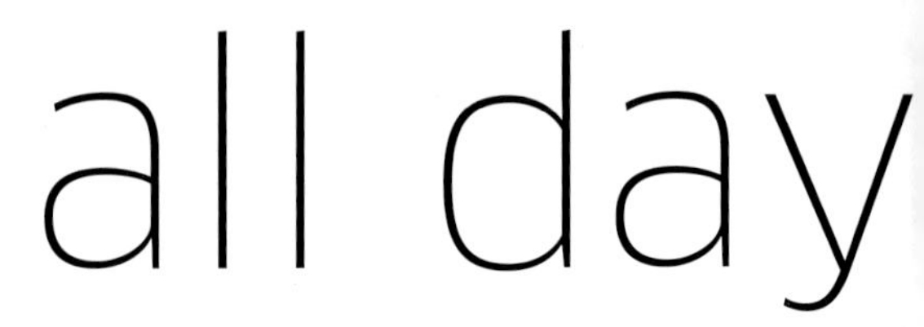

all day

Most people save foreplay until just before sex. Try a different approach: Keep him simmering from morning 'til night.

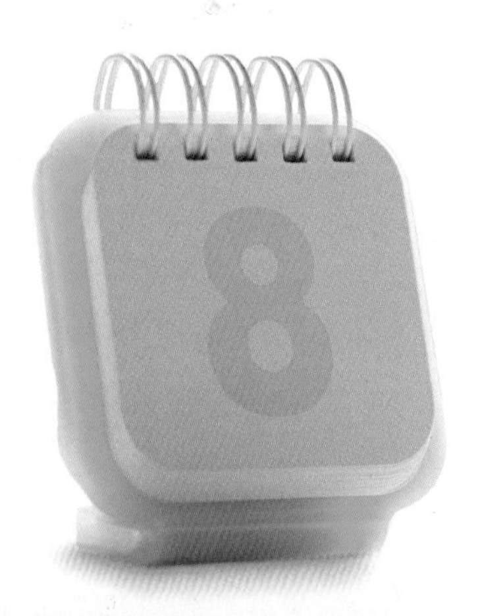

foreplay

Send him **saucy texts or emails** through the day. **Ask questions** that force him to **think about sex.** "Can't wait **to kiss you.** What should I **kiss first**: your **mouth or xxx?"**

Call him when he's **on his way home:** Whisper that you're finding it **very hard to wait.**

naughty wake-up

Coax him into consciousness by sliding your hand around his package. If he responds with a moan of pleasure, get on top and ease him inside you. Move sensually and pick up the speed gradually. It'll be the perfect start to his day. Especially if you make the coffee, too.

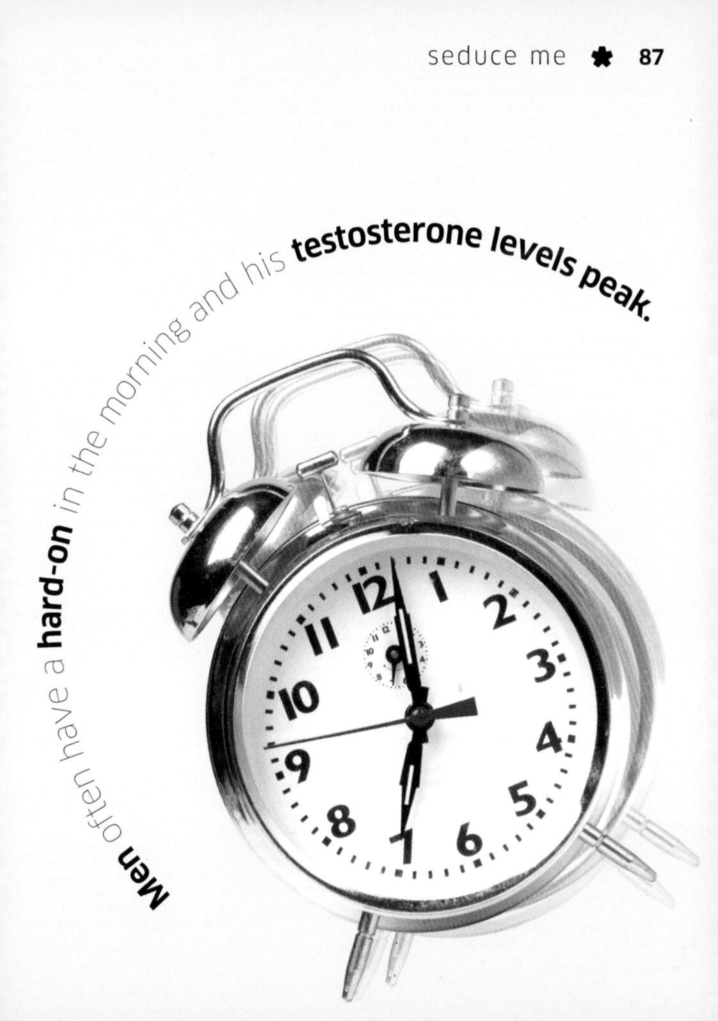
Men often have a **hard-on** in the morning and his **testosterone levels peak.**

show **& tell**

We love when you show us exactly what to do...

* **Show him** how you like to be touched by **caressing yourself. Tell him** when he does it right by **paying him a compliment.**

* **"You're great** with your **hands"** will always **go over well.**

* If you feel **self-conscious, close your eyes** and bask in the **knowledge** that you're delivering the stuff of his **hottest fantasies.**

the first rule of foreplay

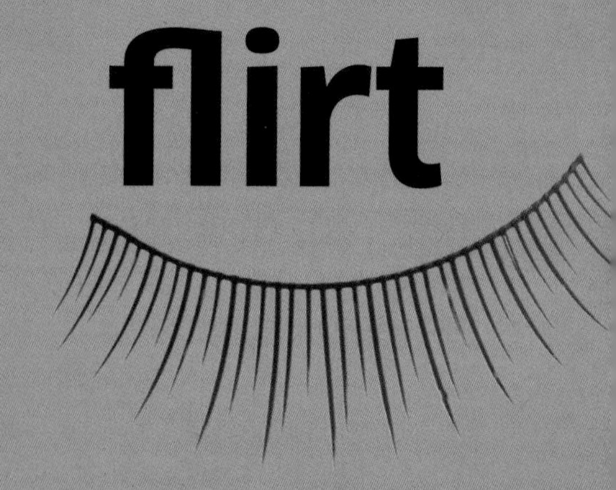

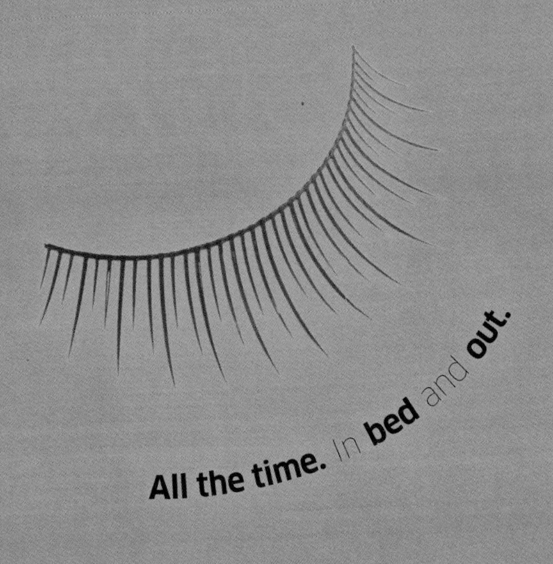

All the time. In **bed** and **out.**

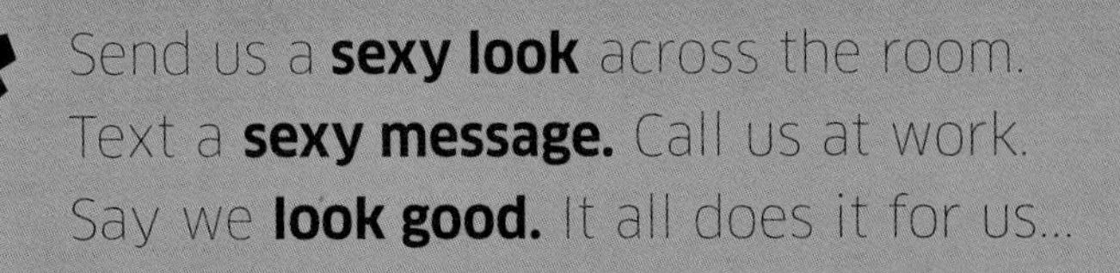

Send us a **sexy look** across the room. Text a **sexy message.** Call us at work. Say we **look good.** It all does it for us...

sexy

There's a trick you can do in any sex position that will boost sensation for both of you:

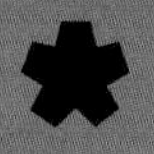

Squeeze him from **the inside** by contracting your **vaginal muscles**. You will both feel a gorgeously tight connection between the two of you. You will also tone up your muscles, which means **stronger orgasms** for you.

workout

✱ Even better, **treat him** to a **pumping action** to make him feel **he's being milked.** Try it just when **he's about to come.**

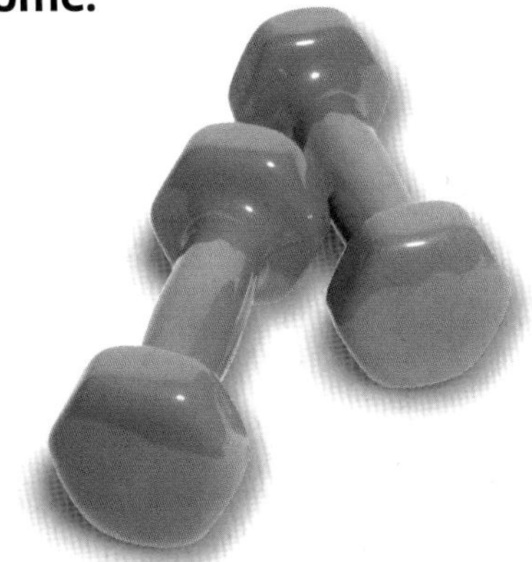

quickies

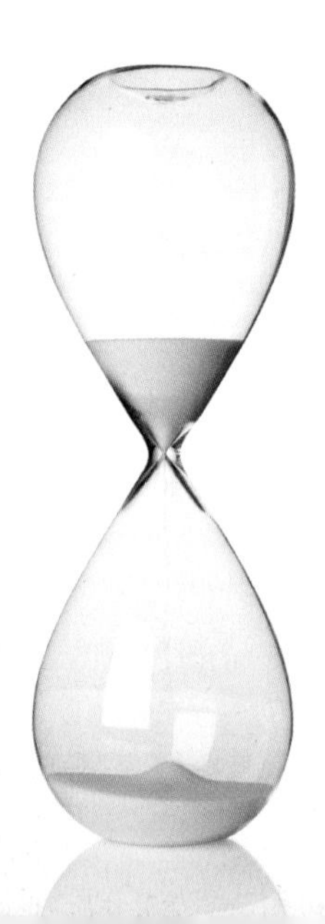

Few men can resist the offer of a quickie. It takes sex right back to basics and feels naughty and animalistic—all things that are guaranteed to launch his rocket.

- Suggest **a quickie** when you've only **got minutes to spare.** Don't bother to **undress**—just drop **your panties.**

- Get him to **stand behind you** for a **stand-up doggie.** Or use the **stairs, desk, or sofa**.

- For an **extra adrenaline rush,** choose a **risqué location** for your **quickie**: an **office, restroom stall, fire escape...**

slowies

Sometimes, we like to take the slow, scenic route. Draw out the tension and build up the desire by taking your time.

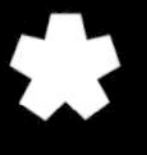

Get steamy in the bath together and then head to a **candlelit bedroom.** Make out for an hour before sex.

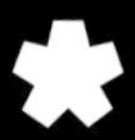

Have him lie on his front and **slowly kiss** the entire length of his body. Turn him over only when he is **shivering with anticipation.**

Spend an afternoon in bed. Stock up with **delicious snacks, champagne, massage oil,** and **sex toys.** Stay in bed for at least **four hours!**

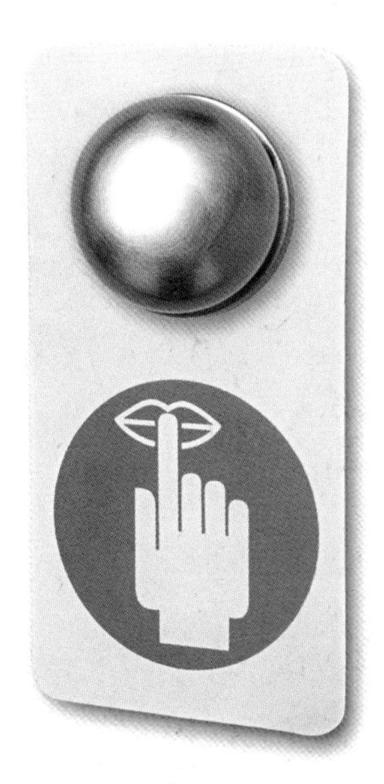

girl on top

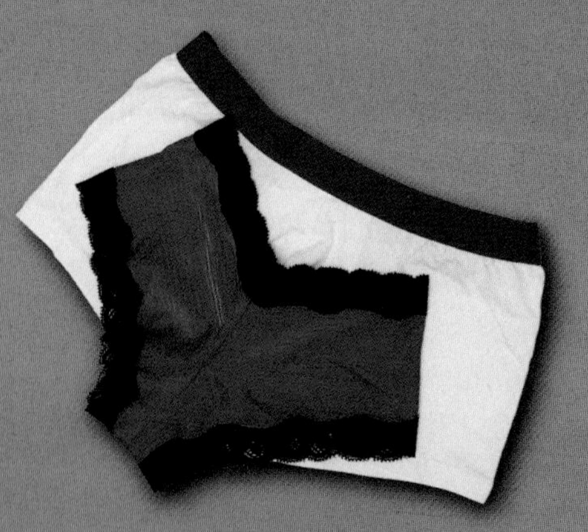

It's the single most exciting position for many men: girl on top. Make him lie back, and climb on top. Now you're good to go.

"I love **seeing her on top:** her breasts, her belly, the **pleasure on her face..."**

"She **comes really easily** when she's on top. That's a **massive turn-on."**

"She **moves her hips** really fast–the friction is **explosive."**

man

We like being on top, too! We like the face-to-face intensity plus thrust control. But if you want to make it more interesting, try these approaches:

Wrap **your arms and legs** around hi koala style. Try a **rocking motion** fo some explosive results.

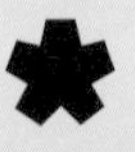

Raise your legs in a large V–it looks **eye-wateringly sexy** and tells him that you're **having a fantastic time."**

on top

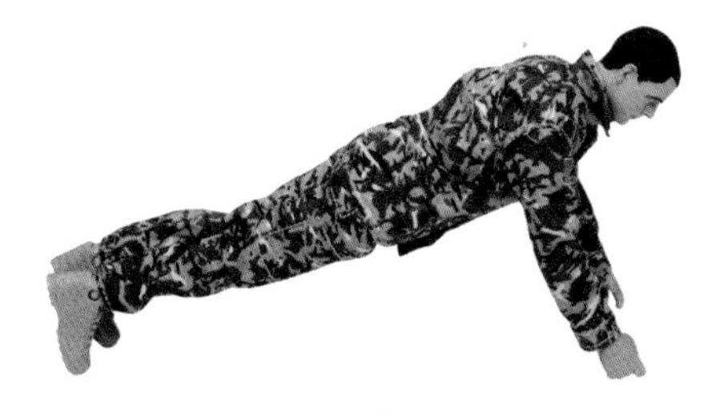

Hook **your ankles over his shoulders.** It's intense, **passionate,** and guarantees **deep penetration,** which should feel good for both of you.

missionary

Want a bit more variety when he's on top? Try some of these missionary twists: Sit on some nice plump cushions or a pillow. This raises you up so we can enter you easily.

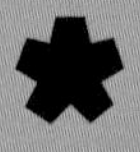

Close your legs once we're in–this **"closing of the gates"** makes everything feel **tantalizingly tight** and gives us **gorgeous friction.**

ary plus

Once in a while, **grab his buttocks** and **pull him in tight** so he can't move. Now **wiggle your hips** and enjoy the **expression on his face.**

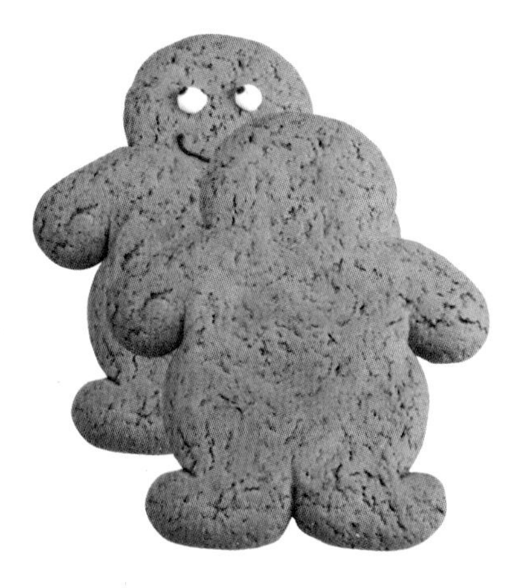

sexy side-by side

Perfect for **lazy Sunday mornings** or lust **late at night, side-by-side** sex is **relaxed** and **intimate.**

Reverse against him in the **spoons position.** Pull him close to you. He'll do the rest.

Or when you're facing each other, **cuddle up** and **kiss. Slide your upper leg** slowly up his **calf and thigh** until it **wraps around his waist.** You are both now in position for **side-by-side action.**

take

For sheer raunchiness, nothing beats sex from behind. We adore the view, too: Just the sight of you sends our lust levels soaring.

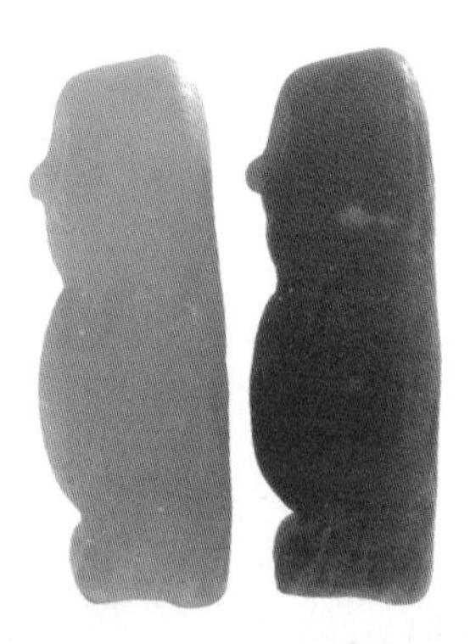

from behind

Choose whether **you want to stand, kneel,** or **lie down.** If you want to try **all three in one go,** start in the **standing position!** It's probably best if you are both **super-aroused**—slipping easily inside is a moment of peak joy. A few **sexy undulations and wiggles** from you send sensations back up the line.

standing

Stand-up sex says one thing to us: You've got to have us right here and right now. So if you initiate a bit of vertical passion with your man, he'll feel like the most wanted man ever.

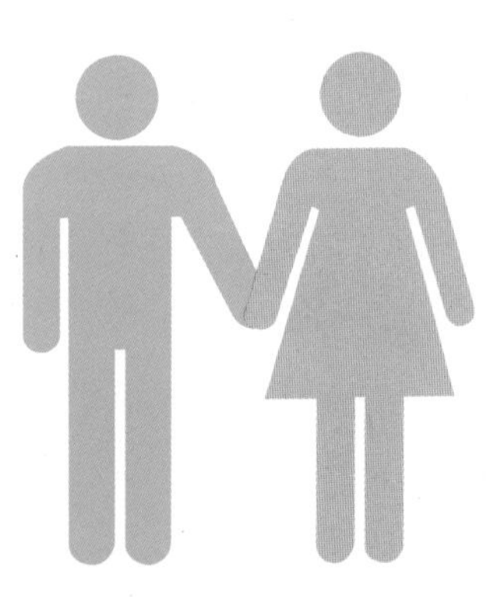

room only

* **“We were upstairs** at a party. She leaned **against the wall** and pulled me close. **I didn’t last very long…”**

* “She **faces the wall** with her hands raised above her in a way that says **‘frisk me.’** It’s pretty exciting and my favorite-ever sex position.”

slinky

Women are often more supple than men, and you can thrill us by bending into an amazing new position that's never even crossed our minds.

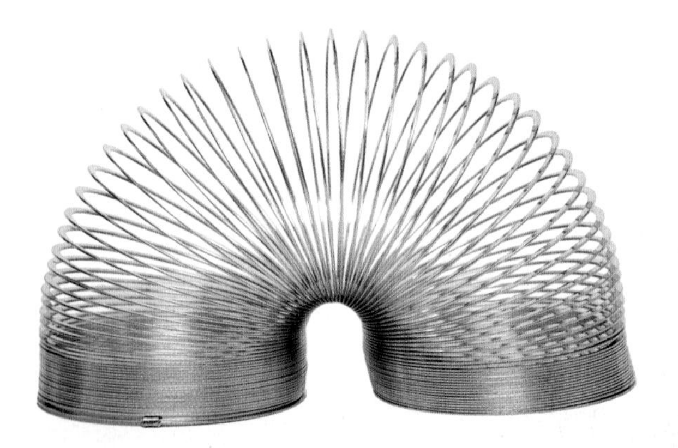

sex

✱ Use a **pillow or sex wedge** to lift you up into **new back-bending positions.**

✱ You know the **position** where he **picks you up** and you **wrap your legs** around **his waist?** Take it further by **leaning back** until **you're inverted** in a backward **handstand.**

✱ **Straddle him** when he's **lying down,** then gradually **lower your body** until **your head** is between his feet.

care for a seat?

Sitting-down sex checks off lots of boxes for men: It feels lusty and we love the face-to-face kissing and the feel of your breasts against us. You get to be in charge, too.

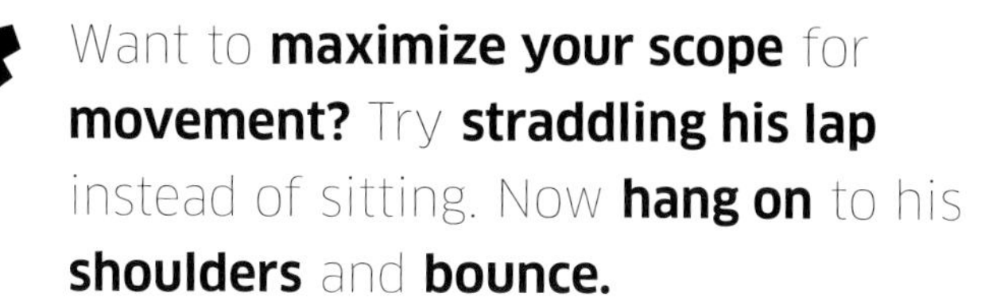

Want to **maximize your scope** for **movement?** Try **straddling his lap** instead of sitting. Now **hang on** to his **shoulders** and **bounce.**

For a **raunchy twist,** sit with your **back to him.** Hold his **knees** for some extra **leverage.**

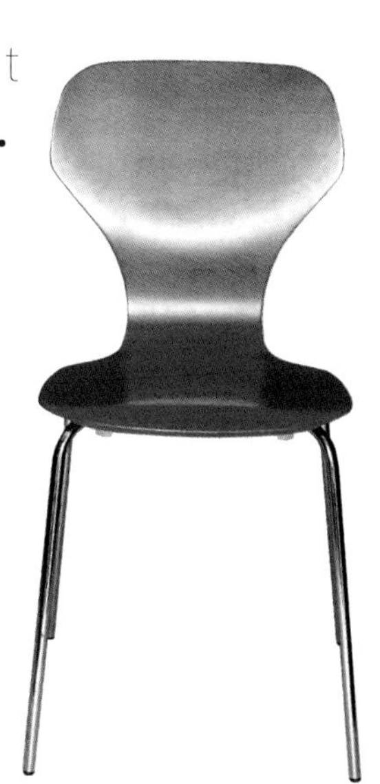

The **sofa, kitchen chairs, rocking chairs, swings,** and **yard furniture** would all work **just fine.**

orgasm

If you want to give us a firecracker orgasm, here are a few tricks to keep up your sleeve:

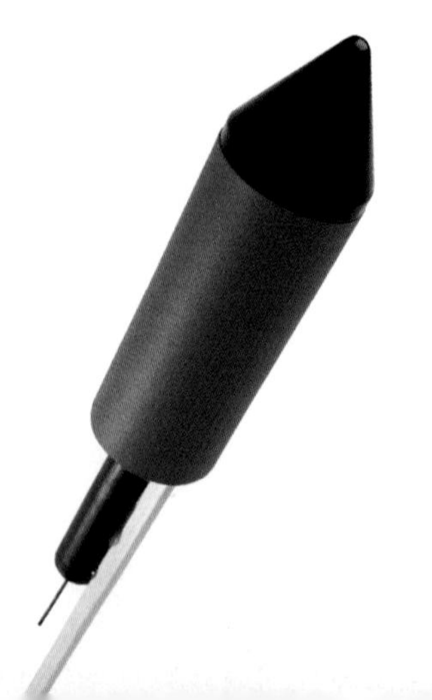

Tip: use sparingly for a "wow" effect.

boosters

- "When I'm just **about to come**, she **slides** her hand **between her legs** and makes a **V shape for me** to thrust through. It feels **amazingly tight.**"

- "She **surprises me** with a hard **spank on my butt**—the shock is **delicious.**"

- "She **presses** on a **spot** just in front of my anus. **It's incredibly erotic.**"

kitchen

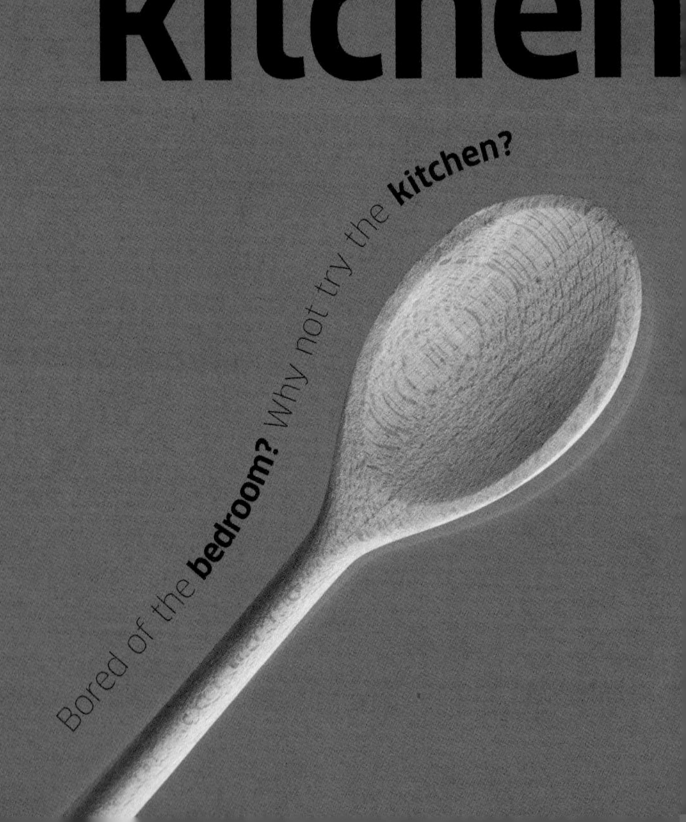
Bored of the **bedroom?** Why not try the **kitchen?**

sex

We **love the idea** of sex on a **kitchen counter:** Standing up and doing **something a bit different** is all good to us. And because we've got our **hands free,** we can put them **to good use on your breasts.**

Get us **into the kitchen** by saying you **"need our help."** Then when you're up on the counter, **open your legs** as a **naughty invitation.** (Of course **you forgot** to **wear panties.)**

steamy bathroo

Bathrooms are great places to get dirty. Whether it's a case of wandering hands in the bath or stealing away for a quickie behind a locked door, the bathroom is tailor-made for sexy, steamy wickedness.

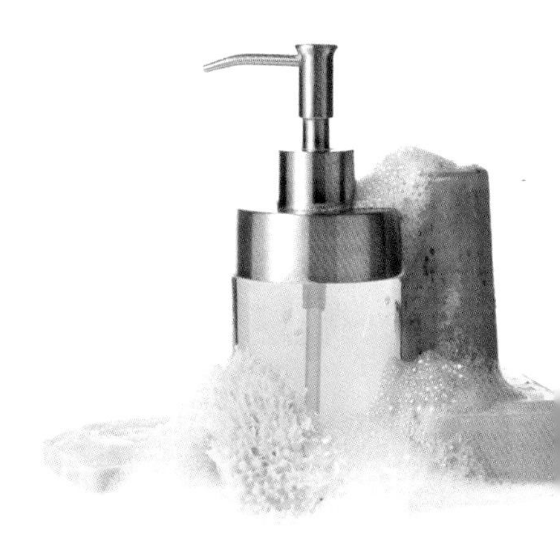

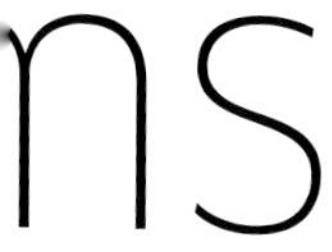

- **Lean on the sink** as he **takes you** from behind. Run the cold water for some **sexy splashes**.

- Share an **erotic bath:** Massage each other with **bath oil,** and tickle each other with a **vibrating rubber duck.**

outdoo

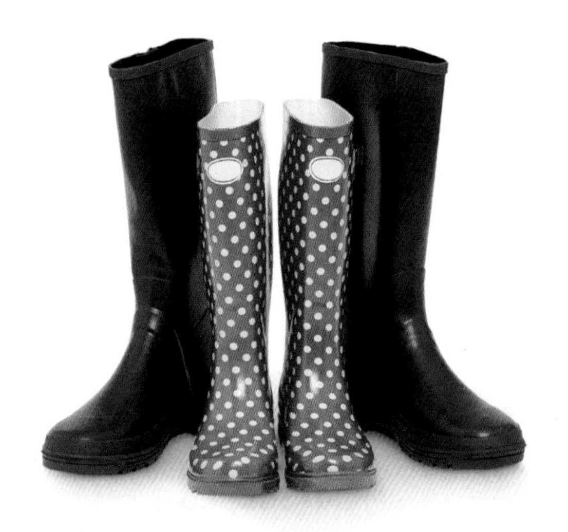

ies

Doing it outside feels, well...earthy. Maybe it's the novelty, the fresh air on our man parts, or the idea of getting caught...

"We had **sex under a tree** in a **park.** We were **taking shelter** from the rain and **got carried away."**

"We found a **secluded bit of beach, covered ourselves** with a **blanket,** and did our **best to be discreet.** An occasional **moan slipped** out, though."

girl

It's often up to men to do most of the in-and-out work during sex. But girls ca be great thrusters, too. And you don't have to be on top. Next time you are in the missionary position, try these tips:

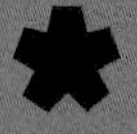

Tell him to **hold himself still** in a push-up position. Now raise your **hips off the ground** and **rapidly vibrate your pelvis.** Imagine your hips are **motorized.**

power

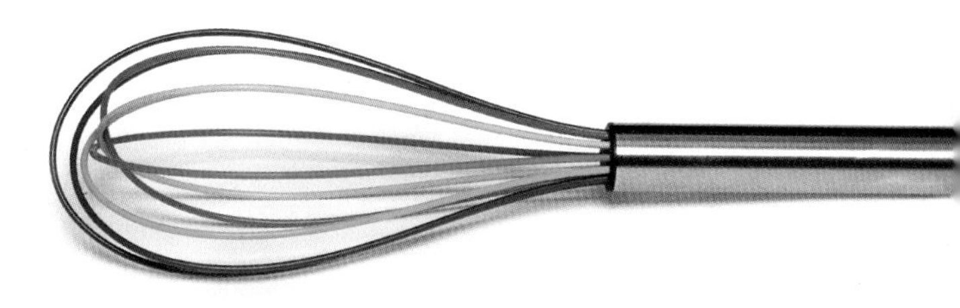

Try **rotating your hips,** too (this time **imagine you're whisking him).** He'll **love the sensation**. In fact, **don't be surprised** if you accidentally **shake an orgasm** out of him.

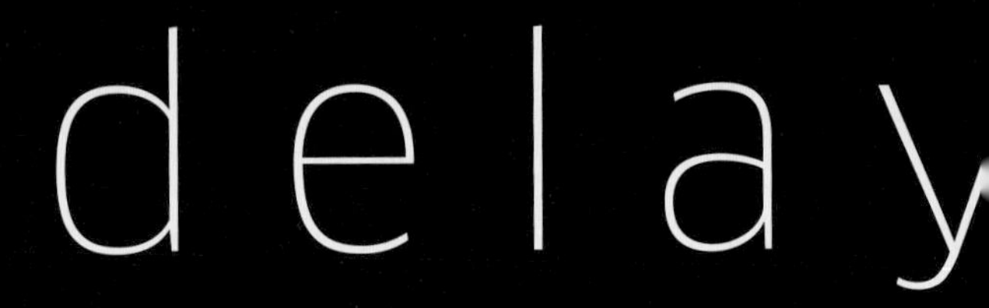

It's happened to all men: We think we've got everything under control and then suddenly—POP—we've blown our cork. Here's how to stop that from happening before you are truly ready:

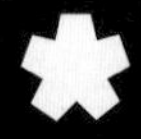

Try **tugging his testicles.** Yes, really. It's fine to just **reach down** and **pull his balls** gently **away from his body** Do it when you sense he's **reaching the point of no return.**

tactics

* Distract him by **firmly massaging** part of his body—his thigh, his back, or his shoulders. **Anything to take his mind off his penis.**

* Suggest a **midsex break—**it's a perfect opportunity for him to **go down on you.** Everyone's a winner!

not

Sometimes we just need a **little coaxing** or a **helping hand.**

in the **mood**

"**She curls up behind** me in spoon position and gently **strokes me.** Even when I'm tired, **it's hard to resist.**"

"**She takes me to bed** and **massages my neck** and shoulders. Then she **kisses** her way **down my back.** By the time **I turn over** I've usually got the **start of an erection.**"

time fo

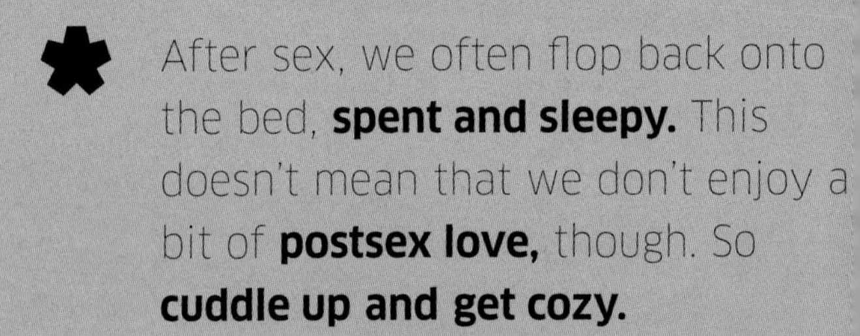

✱ After sex, we often flop back onto the bed, **spent and sleepy.** This doesn't mean that we don't enjoy a bit of **postsex love,** though. So **cuddle up and get cozy.**

✱ Spend some time in bed together. Share a **snack after sex.** Spoon-feed each other your **favorite ice cream** or pop **chilled grapes** into each other's mouths. Think of it as **fuel for round two.**

dessert

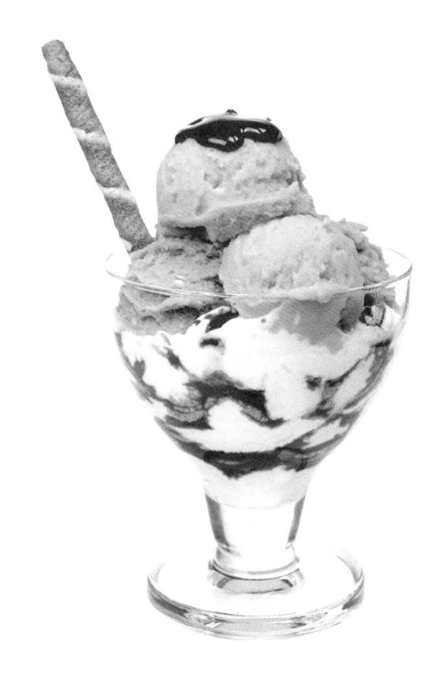

ple

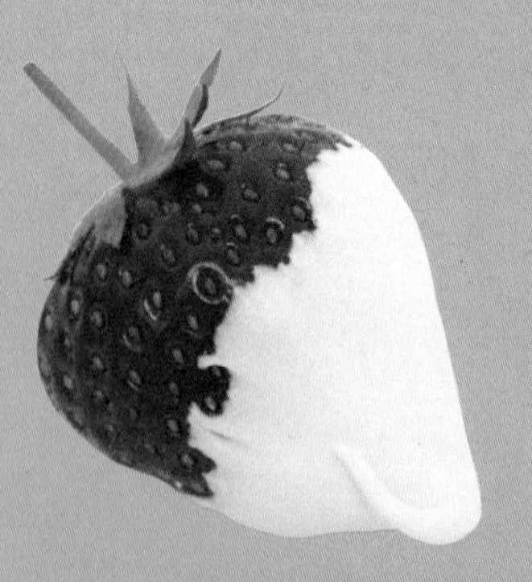

ase
me

dice

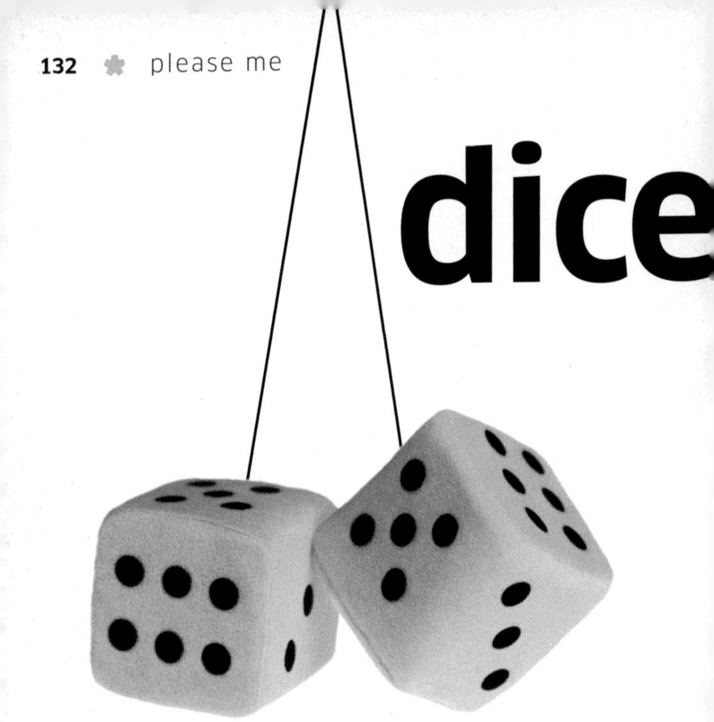

Surprise us. Treat us to a night of unpredictable passion with this sexy game of chance.

game

* Take a **pen and paper** to bed. Both write down **three** of your **favorite positions.** (Feel free to debate the **pros and cons** of each.) **Number** them **1 to 6. Throw a die** to decide which one **you'll try first.**

* Let the die make other **sexy decisions,** too: **which room** to have sex in, **what you'll wear,** what kind of role-playing you'll try, what **sex dares** you'll do, or **how many orgasms** you'll have.

bubbly sex

Don't wait for a special occasion to seduce us with a bottle of bubbly. Why not have decadent champagne sex just for the hell of it?

✱ **Straddle him** with a **champagne glass** in **your hand** and a **naughty look** in your eye. Give him a **"fizzy" kiss:** touch lips and let **champagne trickle** slowly into his mouth.

✱ Take another sip, then **slide** your **champagne-filled mouth** around **his penis.** Don't worry about spills **(it's just another good reason to lick him)**.

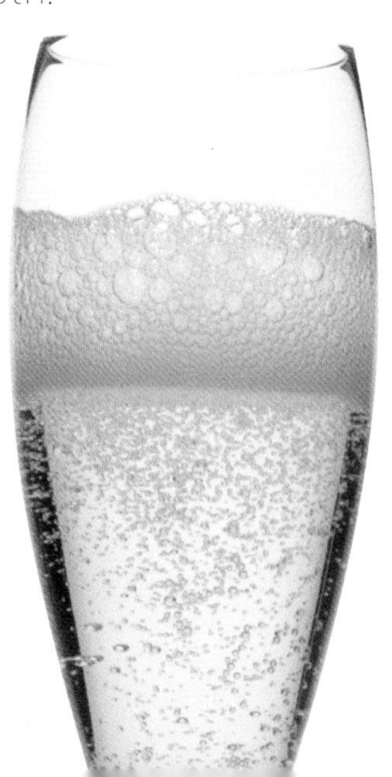

erotic

An erotic photo shoot is the stuff of many men's fantasies so suggest a night behind the camera, with you as the model.

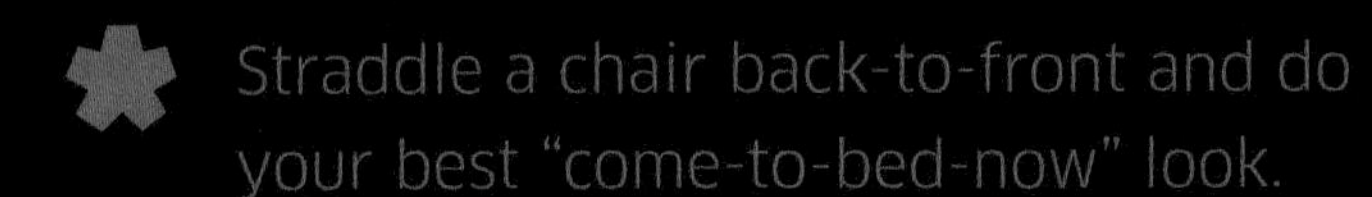

- Straddle a chair back-to-front and do your best "come-to-bed-now" look.

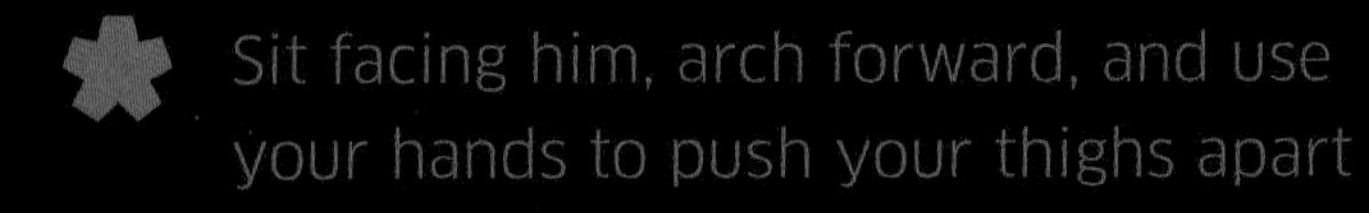

- Sit facing him, arch forward, and use your hands to push your thighs apart

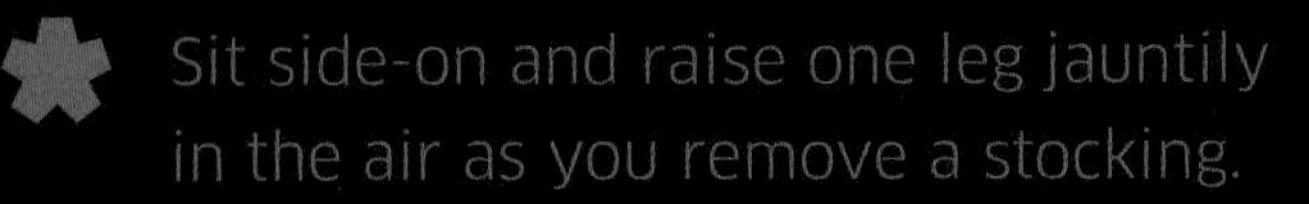

- Sit side-on and raise one leg jauntily in the air as you remove a stocking.

poses

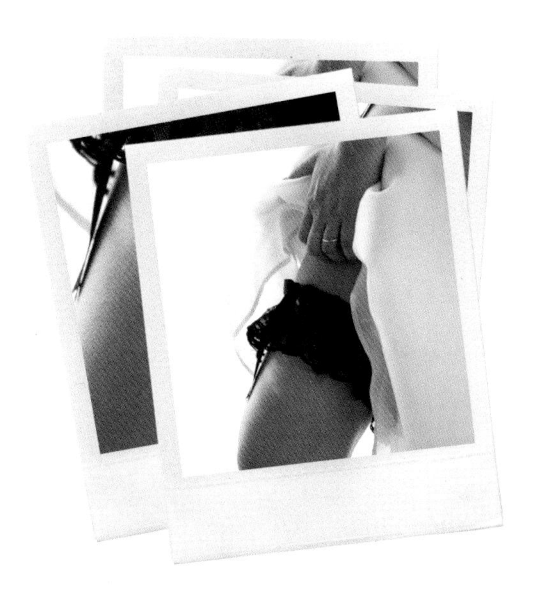

sneak p

Giving us a quick glimpse of your body gets our juices flowing. Even if we don't get to pounce right away.

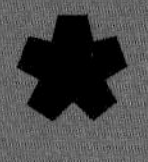

"She wears a short skirt and no panties, then **bends over** as if she is picking something up. She does it to **tease me**—it works!"

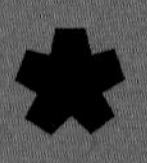

"I love the way her nightie **slips off her shoulder** and shows the **top of her breast** when she's reading."

eviews

"We were having dinner in a restaurant. **I looked down** and her dress had ridden up to show just the **tops of her stockings.** I wanted her **there and then.**"

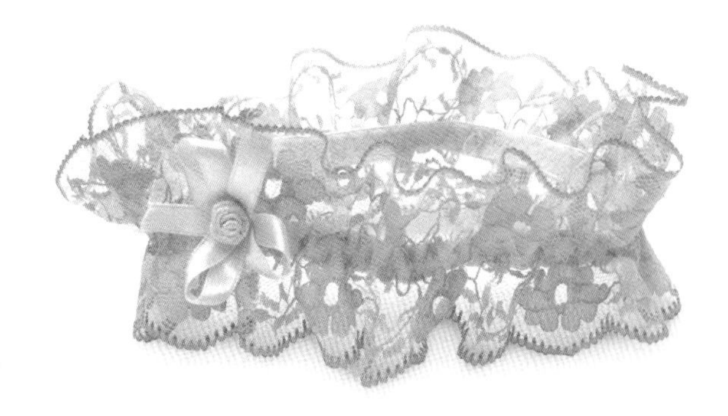

mmmmmmm...

When we're having sex we like to know you're enjoying it as much as we are. That's why we love your moans, sighs, mmmms, and ahhhhhs. They make us feel like experts in the bed department.

* No need to put on a **dramatic stage performance** of **screams, shouts,** and **sobs** that wakes the **neighborhood. Little gasps, groans**, and **ooohs** of pleasure will more than do the job.

* If **you ever feel** driven to **say our name** in a moment of **ecstasy,** our **egos will love it.**

... aaaaahhhh!

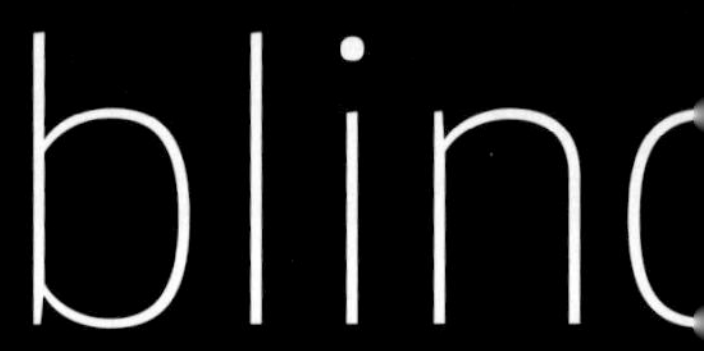

Blindfolds are great sex toys. We put one on, and suddenly you're the one calling the shots. Or wear one yourself, and we get the thrill of being in charge. Either way, everyone's happy.

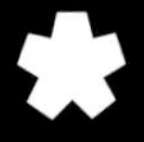

"She **slipped** into the bathroom and **popped a blindfold on me** while I was **taking a bath**. I heard her taking **her clothes off**. Then she was **in the tub** running **soapy hands** all over me. **Gorgeous.**"

old **bliss**

"She was waiting in the bed in nothing but **lingerie and a blindfold.** She told me she was mine to do with as I wanted. It was **incredibly sexy.**"

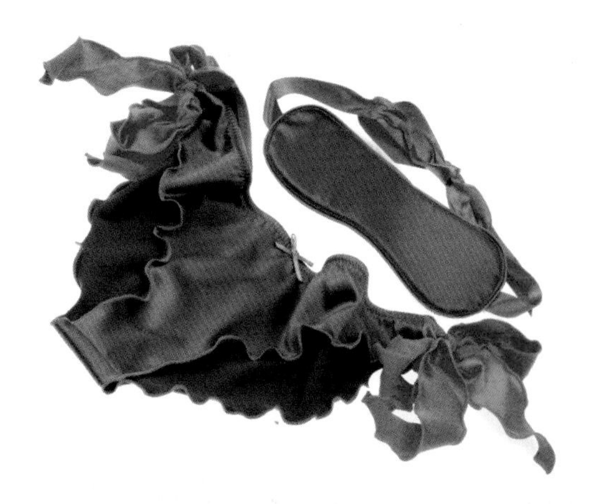

water

We love water. We love being with you in the shower, in the bath, in the hot tub. If you'd like some new ideas, too, how about one of these:

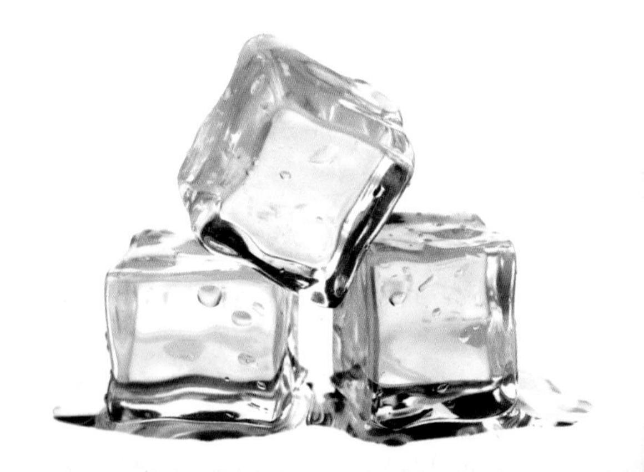

play

✱ Pick the **hottest, sultriest** summer day and drag him into the yard for a **water fight.** Fight over who holds the hose or watering can, and aim to make each other **very, very wet.** Dress code is a **bikini** plus a **tight, white T-shirt.**

✱ On a **hot night,** bring some **ice cubes** to bed to help us cool each other down. We **love the sensation** of cold ice melting against hot skin.

mirror

Watching you at the same time as having sex with you would be a massive thrill. No need for a mirror on the ceiling–one by the bedside will work just fine.

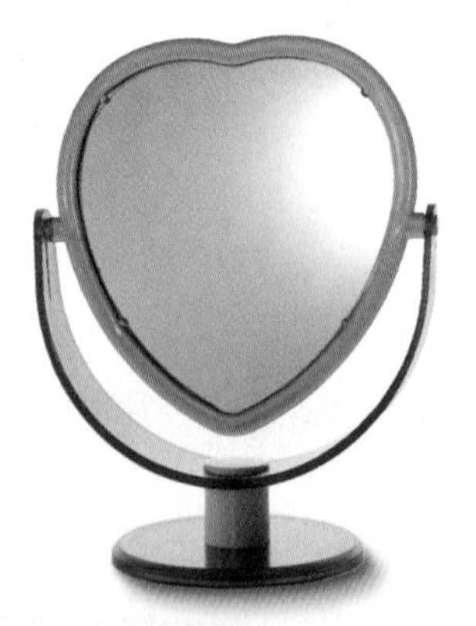

magic

✱ For a **raunchy option,** have **stand-up sex** in front of the **mirror.** He **lifts you up**, you wrap **your legs around**, and he gets to **watch in the mirror.** Or just **bend over** with him behind you. Catch **his eye in the mirror** and give him a wink for added raunch.

sensual

Lots of men get off on sexy hairstyles of the pubic kind. Some of us like the sexy full-grown garden look; others prefer clean-shaven, or a landing strip.

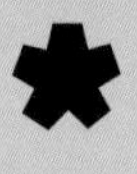

Next time you're sharing a bath or shower, **invite him** to give you a **whole new hairstyle.**

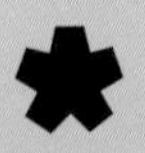

Once he's trimmed you to perfection, ask him to **rub in lotion,** and **seal it with a kiss.**

shaving

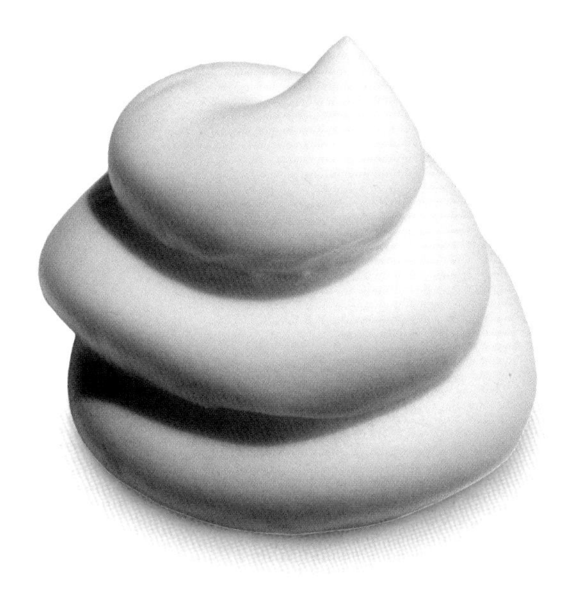

breast

Men love breasts. Fact. We love them in all shapes and sizes. We like to gaze at them, touch, nuzzle, and kiss them. So go to bed and flaunt your breasts for all they're worth. Enjoy the attention we're dying to lavish on them.

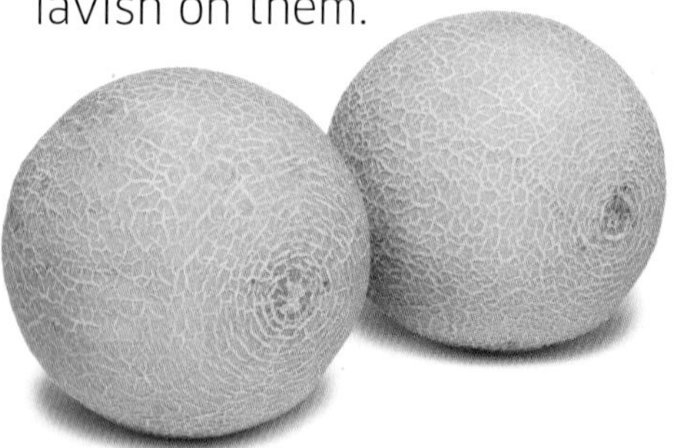

appeal

✱ **"I love it** when she leans over me so I can **feel her breasts** on my face."

✱ "She **makes me watch** while she **drizzles massage oil** all over **her breasts.** Then she asks me to **rub it in.** It's a **massive turn-on."**

✱ "When she's **giving me a blow job**, she sometimes pulls away and **slides her breasts up** and down my body. **It drives me crazy."**

brilliant bu

Feminine and very sexy, the idea of burlesque intrigues us. Dress in **stocking** **heels, snug lingerie, and feathers,** then **shimmy seductively** to your favorite music. Tease as you **slowly undress.**

esque

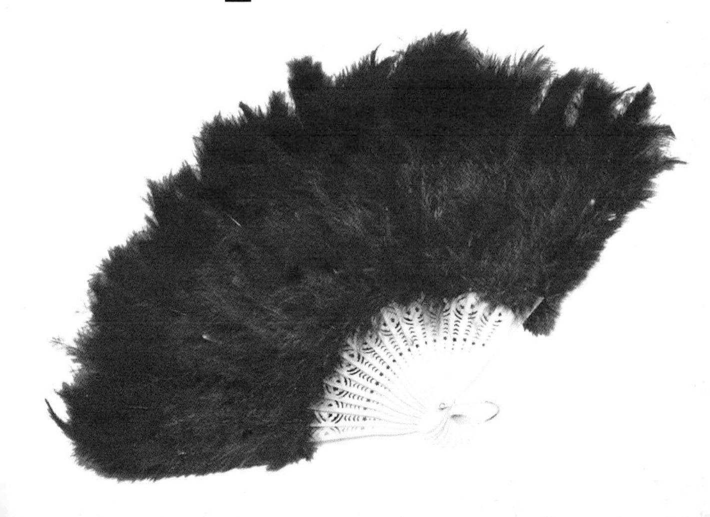

condom techn

The condom moment: It can fill even the most red-blooded man with dread. We worry we'll put it on the wrong way or our erection will wilt or... something. If you can lend a hand to smooth the process, we'll be very happy indeed.

ques

Be the **mistress of condoms:** Pack him **in rubber** so fast, he barely knows what's happening. **Practice** on a **sturdy cucumber.**

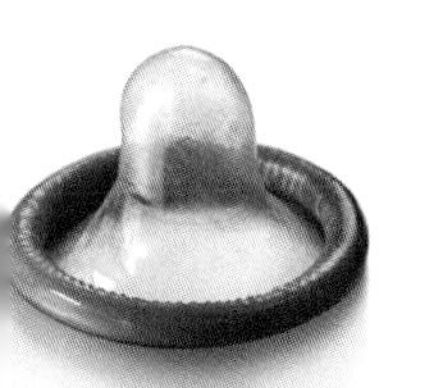
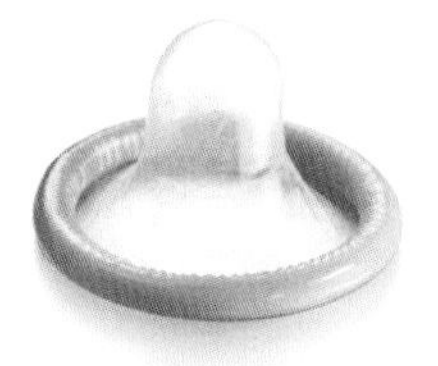
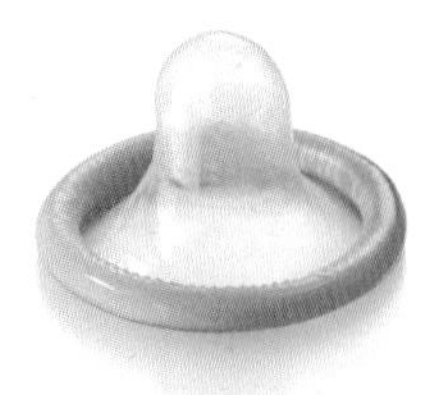

to-do

Use your imagination to make everyday life erotic. Email him a to-do list with a twist. Instead of chores, fill your list with exotic tasks for the night ahead.

8pm: Stroke my naked body with a feather.

ist

9.30pm Blindfold me, then feed me treats.

9pm: Tie my wrists and iss me all r.

10pm: Make love to me!

your

Thanks to cell phones, sexy fun doesn't have to stay in the bedroom—or even the same town or continent. Sex is now possible anywhere. Think of the phone as your hottest new sex toy.

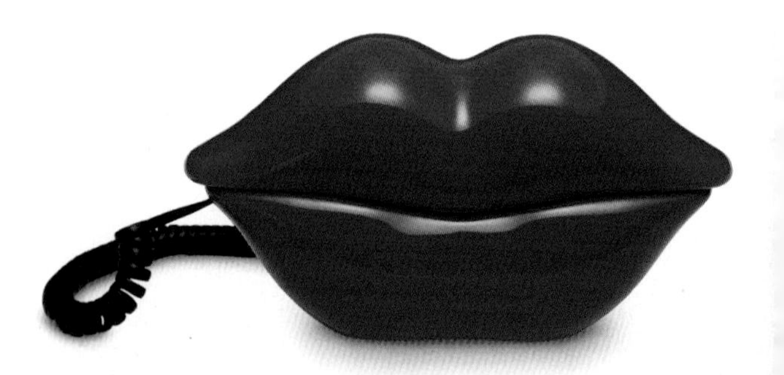

call

Give him a **sexy call** when you're **apart and yearning** for each other. Tell him how much **you're missing him** and how much **you want him.**

Say what you're doing **(lying in bed)** and what you're wearing **(nothing).**

Ask him to **imagine your lips** against **his body** and how you'd take him in **your mouth.** Then you can **both get busy** with **your hands...**

come

We like to see your breasts, face, legs... actually, all of you. So we love it when the lights are left on. If a bright room gives you that "too-much-attention" feeling, candles work, too.

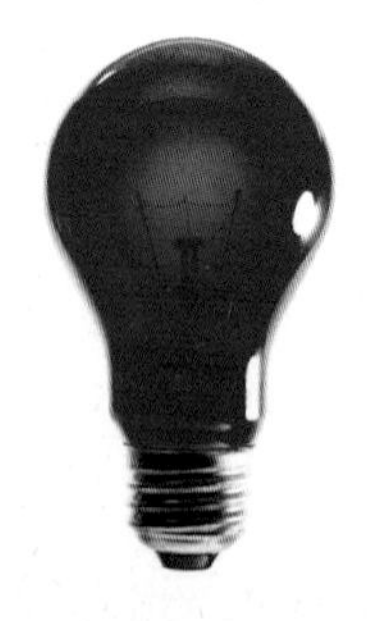
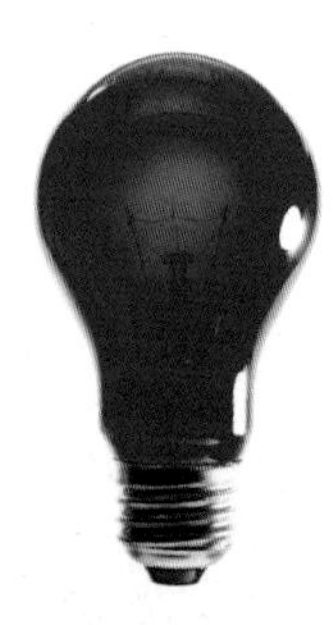
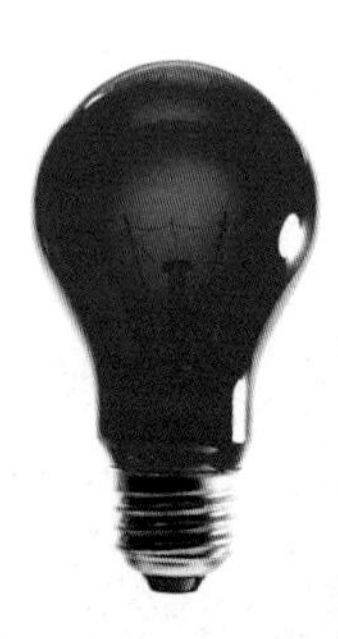

to light

For a **kinkier vibe,** exchange the usual bedroom **white lightbulb** for **a red one.** Suddenly **sex seems a whole lot dirtier.**

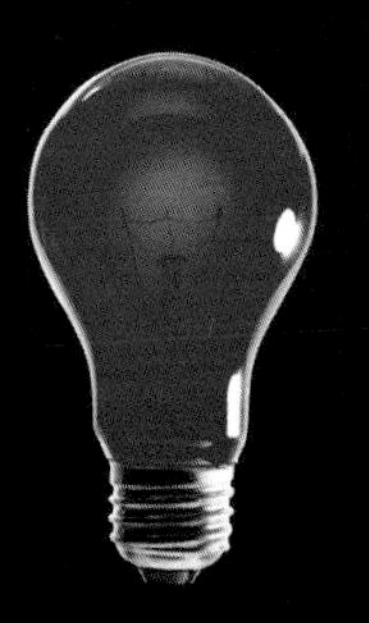
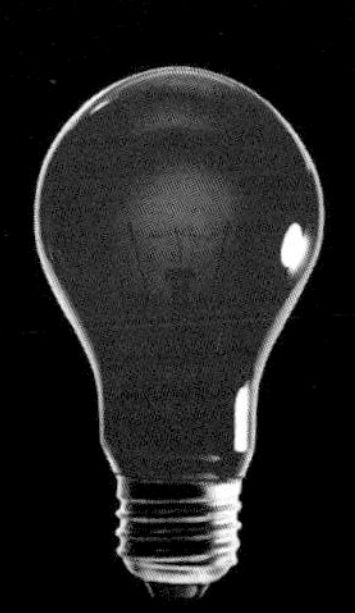
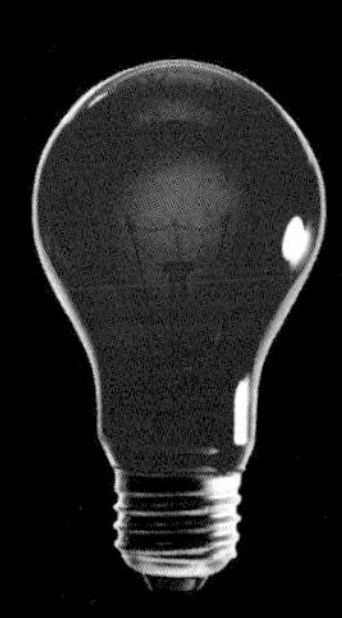

wining &

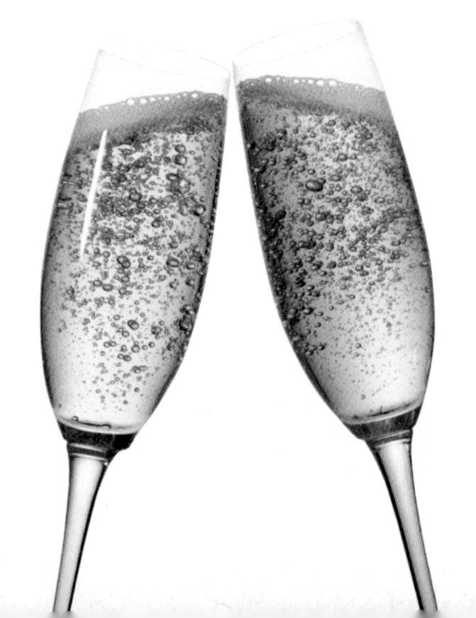

dining

Like you, we love to be wined and dined. It doesn't have to be extravagant. In fact, a simple, sexy meal at home will do just fine.

"I got **home from work** and she handed me a glass of wine. Then she gave me a **handwritten menu.** She'd cooked all my favorite foods. And by **'dessert,'** was the word **'me.'"**

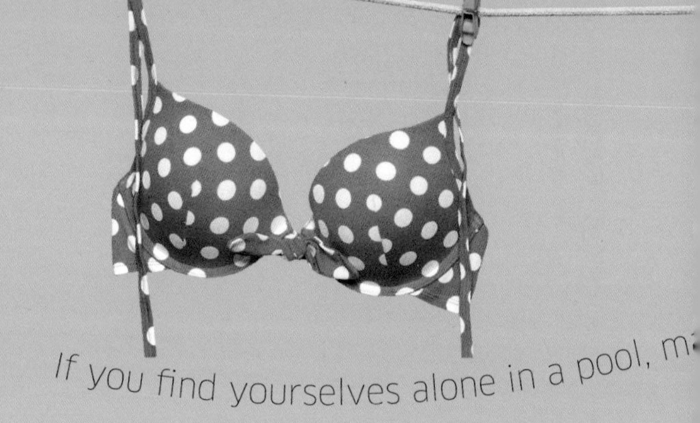

If you find yourselves alone in a pool, m

poo

Make him sit on the pool's edge while you stand in the water. **Slip him out of his trunks** and straight into your mouth.

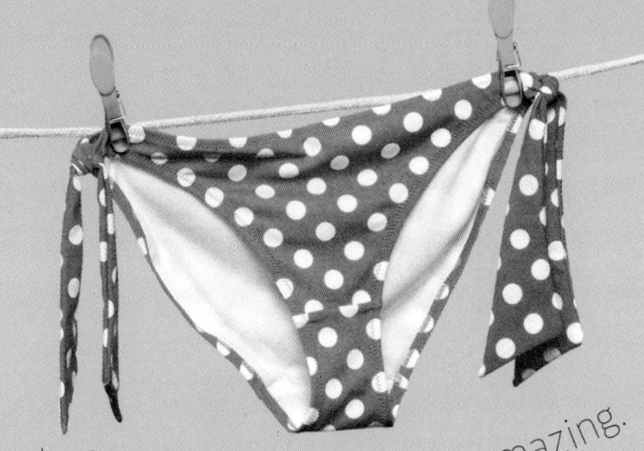

splash. Sex *in the water* feels amazing.

pleasure

When he is ready, he can join you standing in the pool. **Wrap your legs around his waist** for weightless sex.

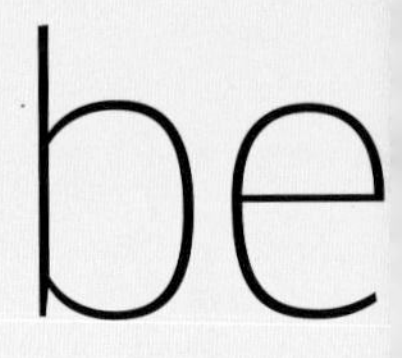

We love it if when you are bold and brazen. Feel free to be in charge and tell us what to do. We are more than happy to become your plaything...

brazen

- Sit him on a chair and tell him **not to move** (tie his wrists to it if you don't trust him).
- Now **take off your clothes,** one item at a time. **Caress** each newly exposed bit of your body.
- Finally, when your panties come off, slip your hand between your legs and masturbate. **Feel free to hop on.**

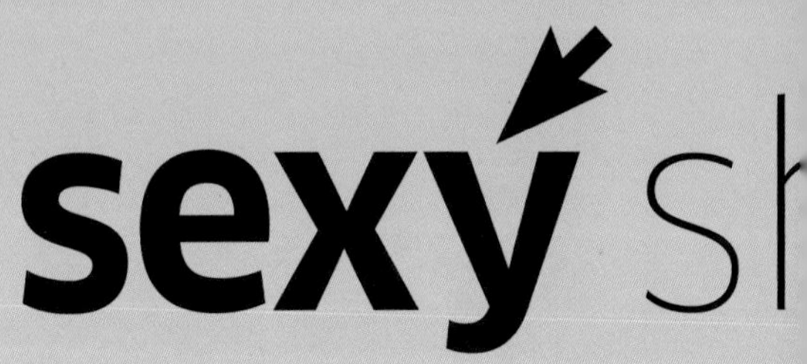

Men and shopping go together like ice cream and pickles. With an important exception: We like gadgets and we like looking at them online. So we'll be quite happy to browse sex toys on a laptop, especially if we're naked in bed with you.

pping

Pretend you're **professional reviewers** assessing the **pros and cons** of each toy. Discuss them in detail, and **buy your favorites.**

If he doesn't know what a particular toy does, say, **"Hmmm, I think** it might do **something like this..."** Offer to **do a demo** with your hands or mouth.

hair

Your hair can give us shivers, tickles, and goosebumps. So tease us with it. Oh, and by the way, we like it when it gets messy...

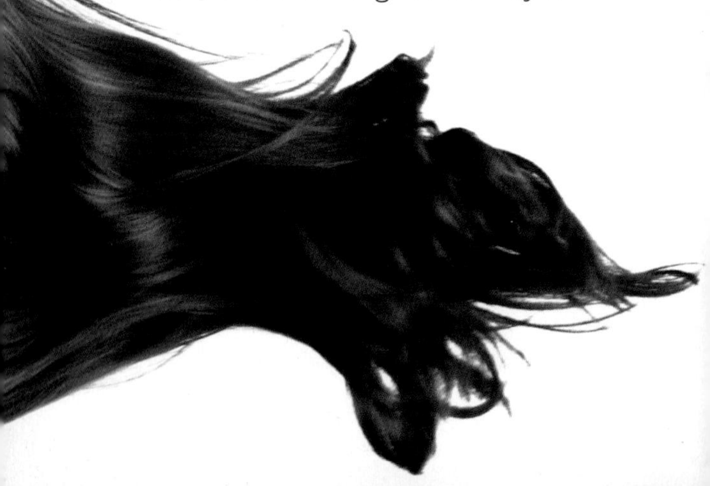

aising

✱ "She sits on top of me naked, then **takes off her headband.** I love that moment when **her hair tumbles** around her shoulders."

✱ "She **winds her hair around my erection** and then pulls slowly away. It **feels fantastic."**

✱ "We have sex in reverse cowgirl and **she arches back** so her hair tickles my chest. **It looks so sexy."**

give him

It seems like girls have lots of fun when it comes to vibrators. We'd love to share in the excitement, so invite us along for a threesome.

a buzz

* **Just watching** will jump-start his desire—give him a **live demo of vibrator play.** Or let him do the work: Let him hold a **vibrator** against **your clitoris** while he's **inside you.**

* Then it's **his turn.** Run it **smoothly up and down** the length of **his shaft.**

material girl

Caress his package through the fabric...

Tease him when he's lying in bed in just a pair of underwear. Trace the outline of his penis and balls through the fabric for an interesting wake-up call.

- **Steam him up** by putting your **lips close** and **breathing hotly.** You can even try **giving his shaft** a very **gentle bite** though the material.

- **Don't even think about** releasing him until he's bursting at the seams.

get

Skip dinner and go to the gym together instead. Exercise gets the blood pumping, the pulse racing, fires up your sex drive, and gives you faster and stronger orgasms.

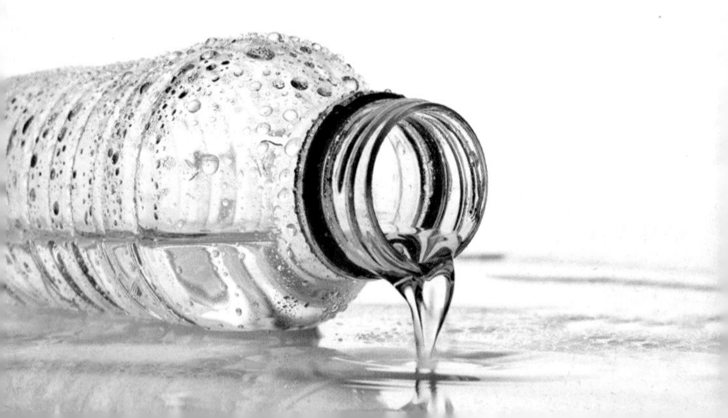

sweaty

- Throw him **flirty looks** across the machines as you **pedal, bend, pump, and push.**

- Afterward, go home and start **smooching while still sweaty.** (The smell of sweat is a total **aphrodisiac.)**

- Now jump into the shower together, **lather up,** and satisfy **your lust** right **then and there.**

movie night

Choose a film that will turn you on. He'll enjoy watching the porn, but the big thrill will be watching you. Set a 15-minute "no touching" rule, and let the tension build up between you.

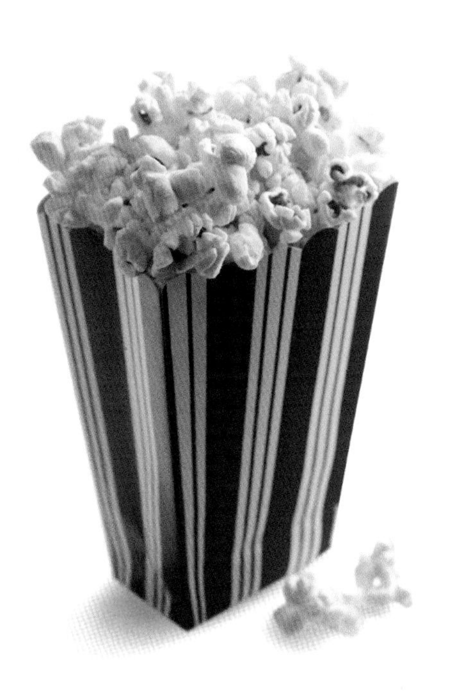

leave your hat on

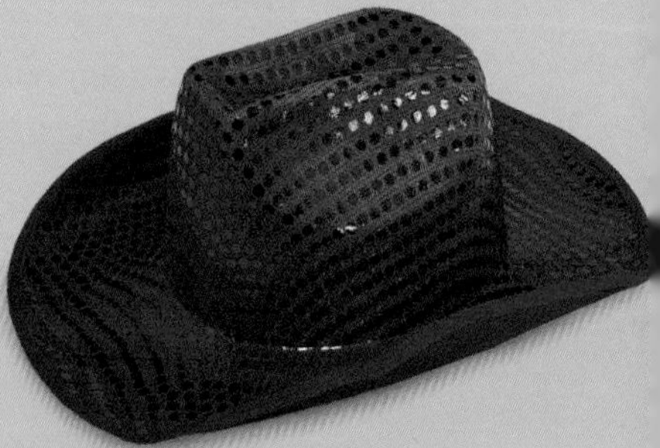

Come to bed in a hat. Sounds weird, but it's a playful, sexy way of telling us what kind of mood you're in. Think of it as role-playing without too much effort.

Try these hats on for size:

Stetson = wild passion
Cop's hat = sexy dominance
Gangster's trilby = naughty and seedy
French maid's cap = flirty and saucy
Nun's headpiece = secretly sinful
Top hat = it's showtime

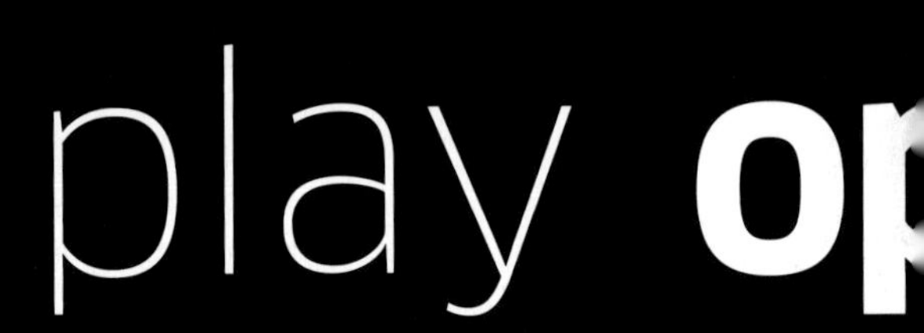

This one's easy. Just do the opposite of what you normally do.

osites

✱ Instead of wearing **raunchy red lingerie,** wear **virginal white.**

✱ Instead of **rose petals** and **candles,** try a **porn film or magazine.**

✱ Instead of **missionary,** try **standing.**

✱ Instead of the **bedroom,** try the **backyard.** And so on...

eastern

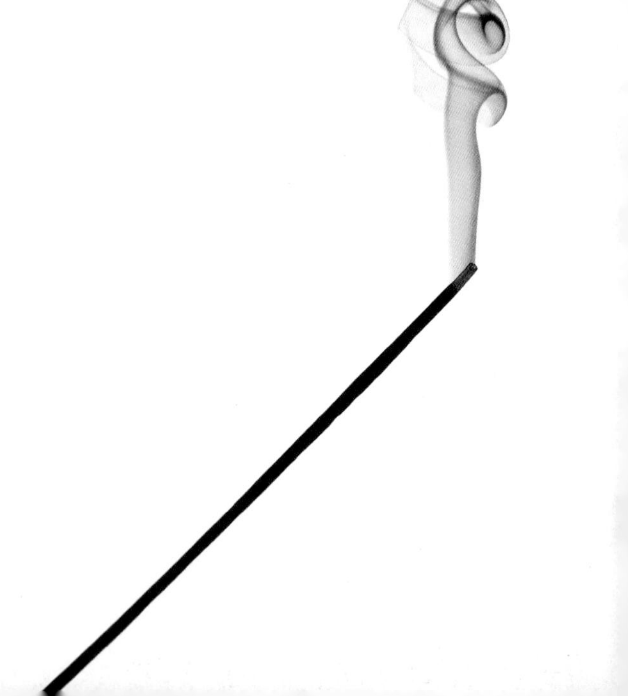

spice

Prove that tantra isn't just about deep breathing: Treat us to a night of blissful Eastern eroticism.

- Fill the room with **exotic musky scents** and **flickering candlelight.**
- Dance together to **slow, sexy, rhythmic music.**
- Take time to enjoy your bodies with **massage, foreplay,** and **slow sex.**

sex by

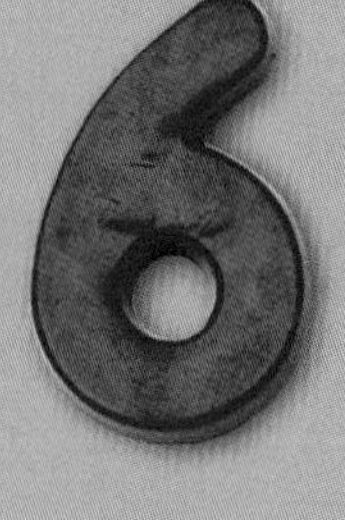

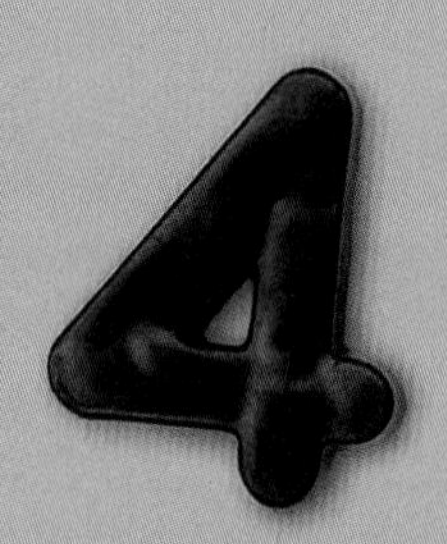

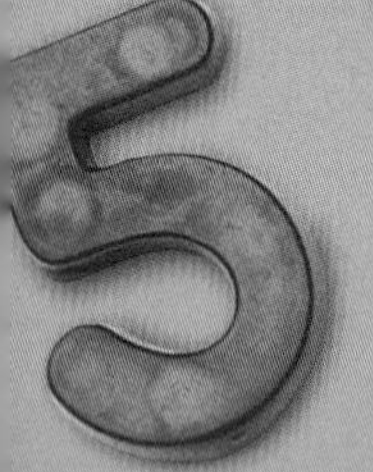

Ever heard of sex by numbers?

numbers

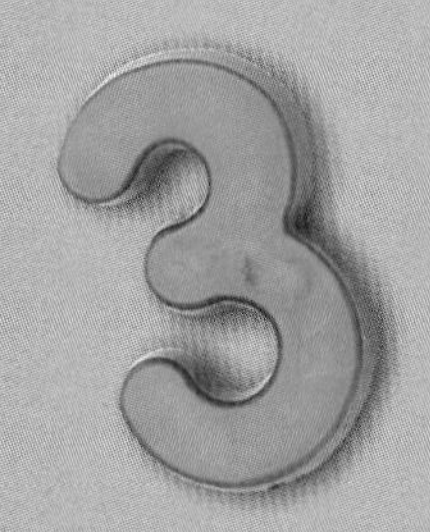

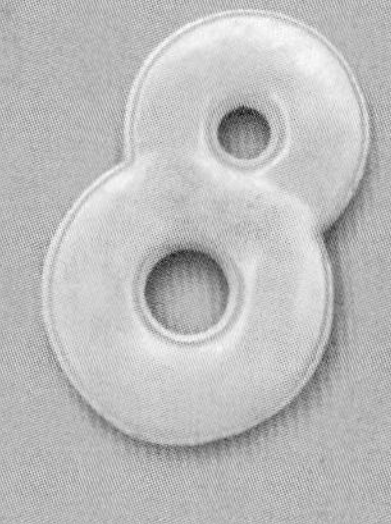

You just write the numbers **1 to 10** on your body in **chocolate body paint** (think carefully about the order). Our job is to follow the numbers as we **lick, caress, and lavish attention** on each part of you, starting with 1 and climaxing—literally—with 10.

G marks the spot

We like the idea of driving you G-spot crazy. The truth is we can't always put our finger on it. Which is why we're happy to lie down with you for a bit of private instruction.

Hand him a dildo. Let him guide it inside you and **shout, "There!"** when you feel a pleasure surge on your front wall. Tell him in **words, moans, or squirms** how you like to be stimulated. Get him to find **your G-spot with his finger–**it should be swollen and **easy to find** by now.

heel

High heel shoes do it for us. Whether it's a pair of killer stilettos or some thigh-high boots, our eyes will be glued to your legs.

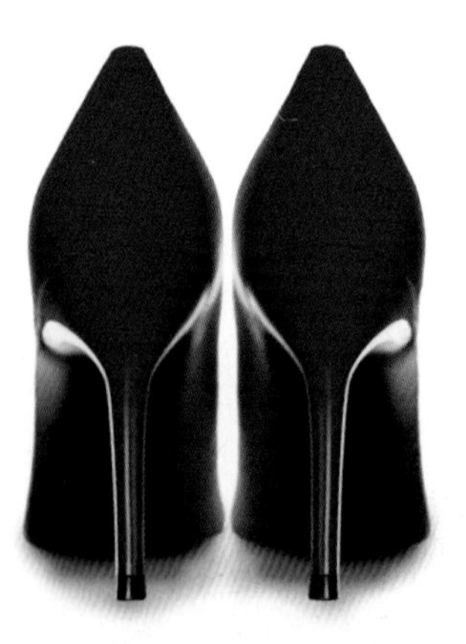

power

✱ "She straddled me wearing **heels and stockings.** Then she slowly moved into a **deep squat** to have **sex** with me. It was **very difficult** to contain myself."

✱ "She called me into the bedroom where **she was lying** on the bed **naked,** apart from a **pair of stunning high heels.** She'd very casually rested her feet up **against the wall."**

dirty

We **love** the sound of your voice, especially when **you sound turned on.** And it's really good to hear you **talking about sex,** rather than everyday stuff.

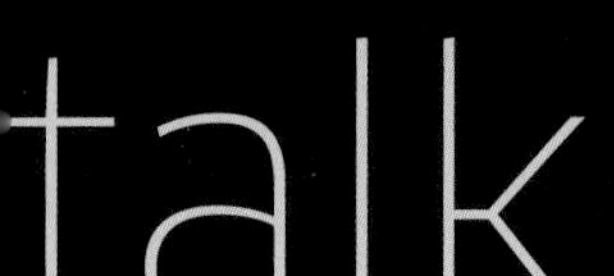

- **Call us at work** or when we're out of town, and speak slowly in your best breathy **"got-to-have-you-now"** voice.

- In the bedroom, **tell us slowly and calmly** what you plan to do or what you want us to do. **We will pay attention, and that's a promise.**

guy comp

Guys like compliments, too. We just like to be praised about slightly different things by you. These three will do nicely:

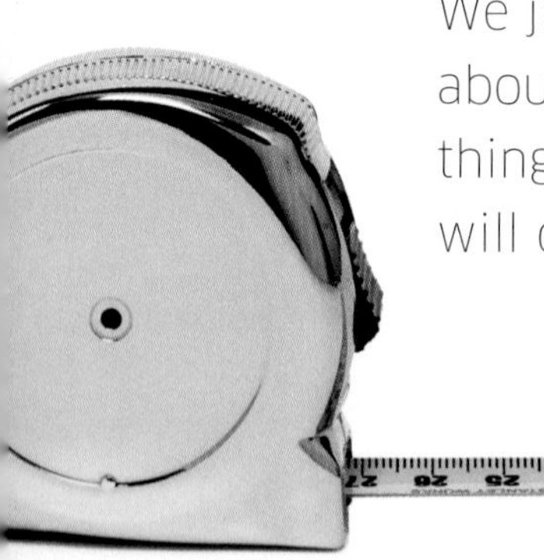

ments

His sense of humor.
His package.
His talents in bed.
(And it will make us very happy.)

working

Office sex...we shouldn't find it exciting, but we do. If you can, sneak into his office for a late night tryst. Try sex on the conference room table, on the edge of his desk, in the elevator, in the supply closet, on the photocopier...

late

Throw in a **bit of power play** to ramp up the **excitement.** You're **the boss** and you're **giving him orders: "Undress now,"** is a good start. Or **he's the boss** and you're the sexy **temp-turned-temptress.**

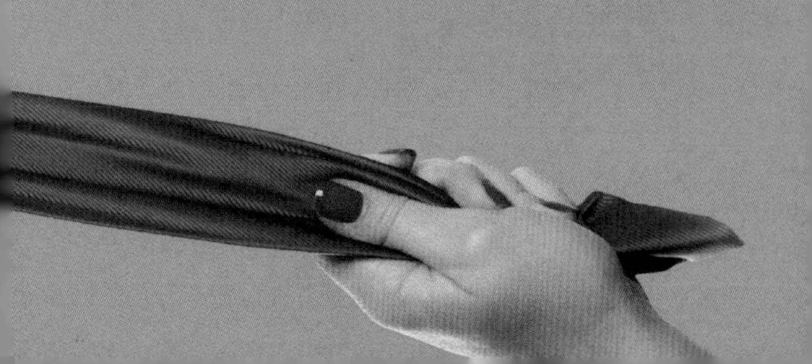

not tonight honey

Sounds crazy, but not having sex can send our lust levels soaring. We're not likely to suggest this ourselves, so it's up to you to take the lead.

"She **booked us** into a **boutique hotel** and said **'no sex'** until then. We ripped our **clothes off** when we checked in."

"She suggested **erotic massage** instead of sex for a week. It improved our **sex life** and relationship."

keep clothes

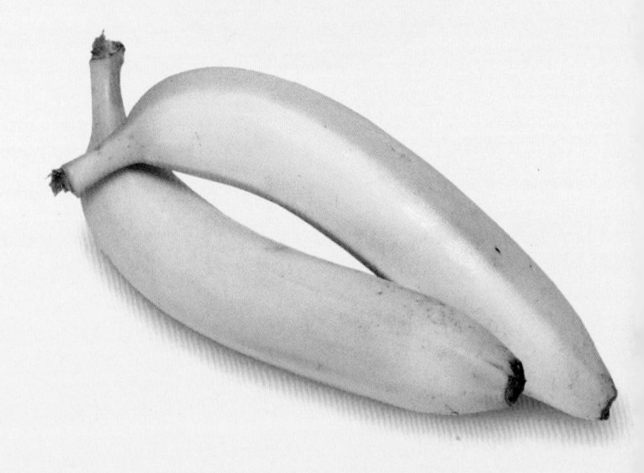

your
on

Remember humping with your clothes on? The teenage lust. The groping and grinding. The frustration! Take us back there. **Treat us to a nostalgic, fully-dressed romp.** There's something explosive about feeling you through fabric. **Ideal when you only have time for a quickie!**

thr

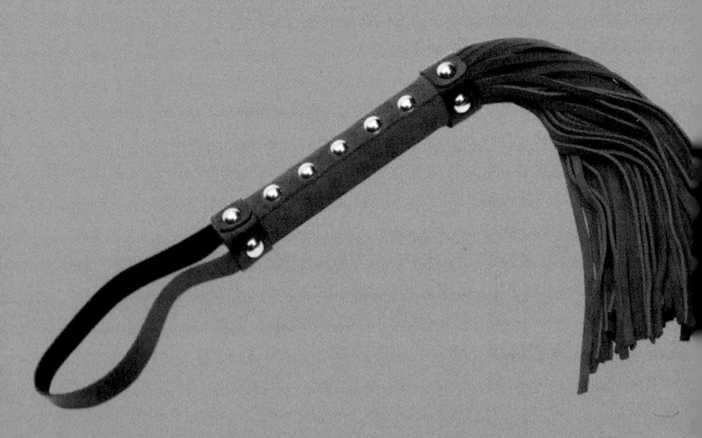

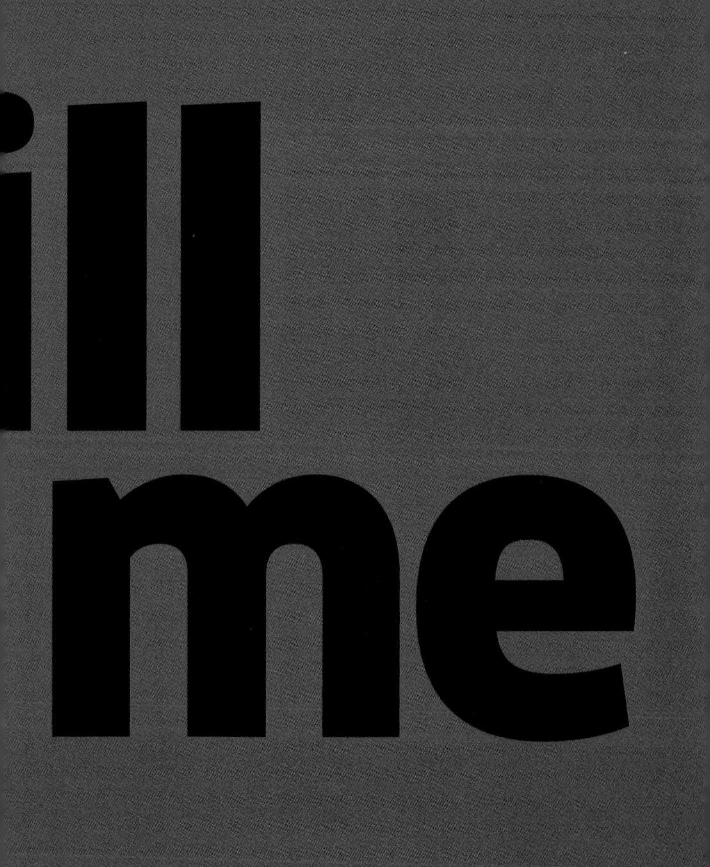
ill
me

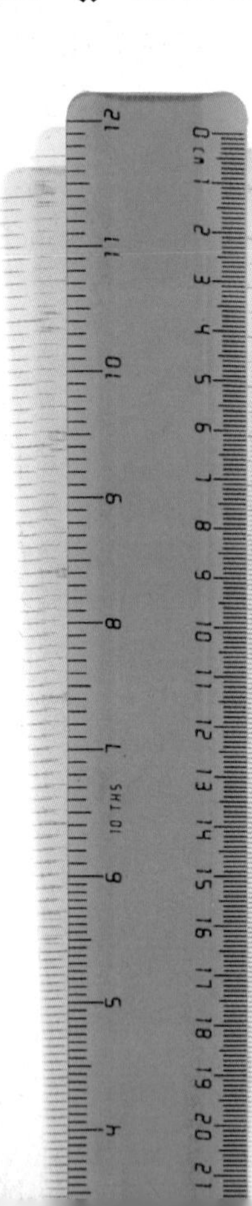

teach

Next time you give him a back massage, throw in a surprise spank. If he gasps with pleasure, you are on to something...

him a lesson

- Spanks send **tingles, stings, and fizzes** of pleasure through **his buttocks** and the **boys in the front, too**.
- Get adventurous with a **spatula or paddle.** Tell him to bend over, then **alternate spanks with soft caresses.**

private

A close-up glimpse of your privates can drive him completely gaga. It doesn't matter whether you're standing, lying, or sitting–as long as your legs are wide open so he can take in the glorious view.

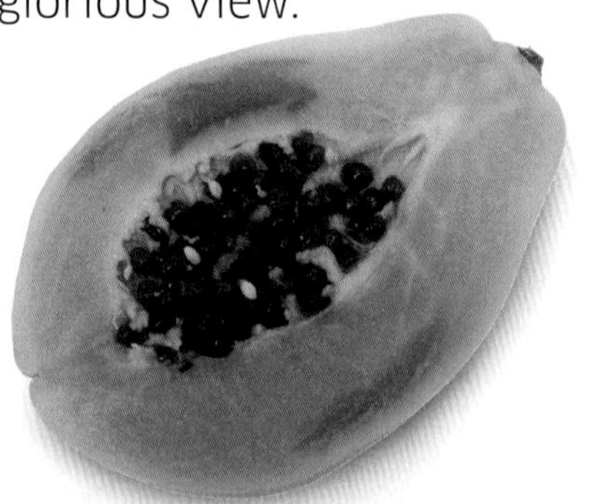

view

"She lay back in bed and used her **fingers to spread her lips.** It was the **hottest invitation** I've ever had."

"She stood with one foot on either side of **my head.** As I looked **straight up her skirt,** she hooked her **panties to the side** with her fingertip."

"I went **in the bedroom** and she was **on all fours** with her **bottom up**—I've never been **so turned on."**

back

It's naughty, it's taboo, and it delivers some hot sensations. These are just some reasons why **anal sex** might be high on his wish list. Despite what you might think, **popping in the back door** doesn't have to hurt and doesn't involve extreme S&M.

door entry

✱ This is best when you are **extremely aroused** so get him to **lavish you with sexual favors first**. Massage lubricant between your cheeks and along his shaft. Take insertion **a little at a time**. Relax your muscles and breathe out as he enters.

chain him up

This is bondage for beginners. No chains or cuffs required—a silk scarf and a coat hook are all you need.

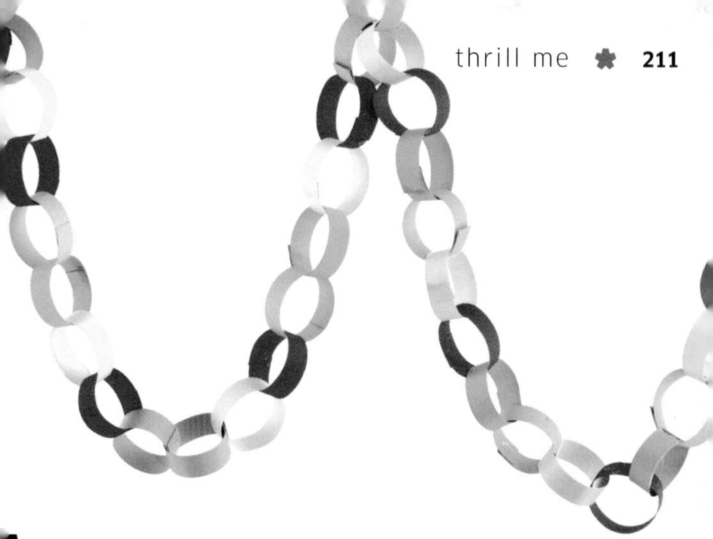

Start both standing up. After a **passionate kiss,** get him to cross his wrists. **Bind them together** with a scarf. Push his hands **above his head** and loop the scarf over a handy coat **hook just above him.** Slink down his body, undo his fly, and take him **firmly in hand** (or mouth).

peep

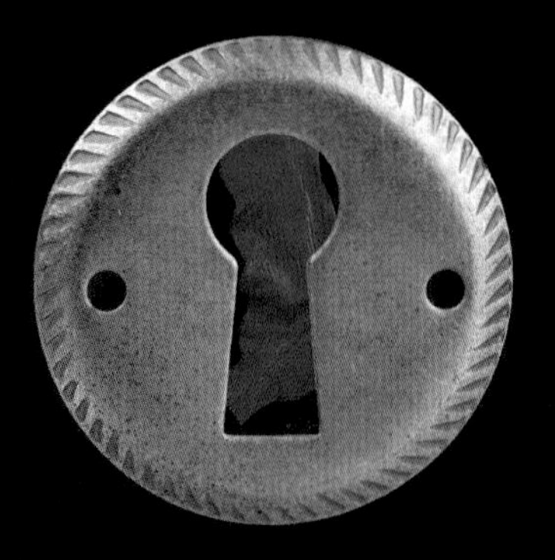

Spying on a sexy scene is a classic schoolboy fantasy. It's also one many of us still love, even though we might not admit it.

show

Indulge him: Set up a scene in which **he's the voyeur.** Leave the **door ajar** when you're **doing something sexy.** Or arrange a **role-play** in which he **peeps through the keyhole.** He then comes in and **ravishes you.**

Great **peep show scenes** include: drying your body after showering, **caressing body lotion** into your naked skin (especially your breasts), and **pleasuring yourself** with a sex toy.

hello

Shake up sex with a scorchingly hot role-play. The plot is simple: You're two strangers meeting in a bar. You find yourselves in the grip of an electric attraction that you just can't ignore...

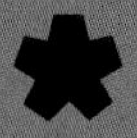

"I hardly recognized her. She had changed her hair and was wearing this mind-blowing dress. **I couldn't believe my luck."**

stranger

"I **love flirting** with her **all over again.** That **thrill-of-the-chase** thing really **gets me going."**

"It leads to **the most amazing sex.** We do things **we'd never normally do.** She gets **very dominant."**

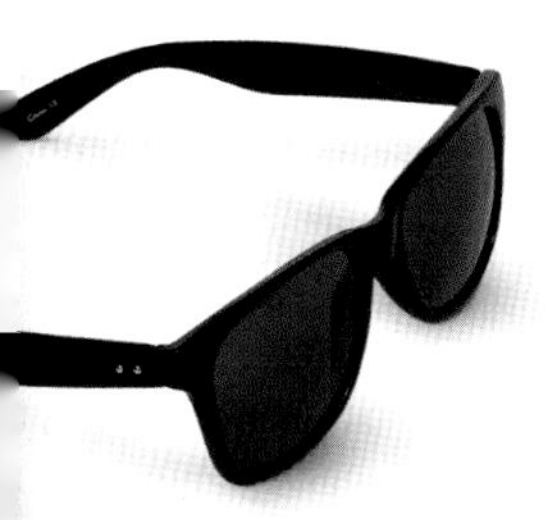

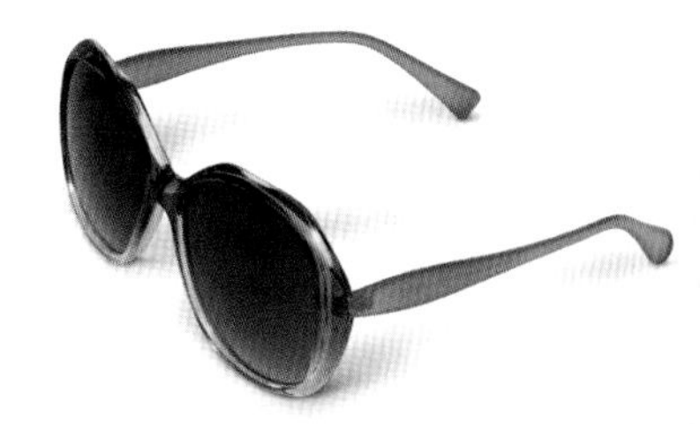

in sus

You know how blindfolded sex works? Taking away sight enhances the other senses. Well, try going a step further: Take away his hearing, too.

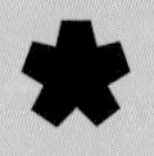

Put a **blindfold on him,** and plug him into **some funky music** on a pair of headphones. Now treat him to a variety of **kinky delights.** The suspense alone will keep him excited. **Kiss, lick, and nibble.**

pense

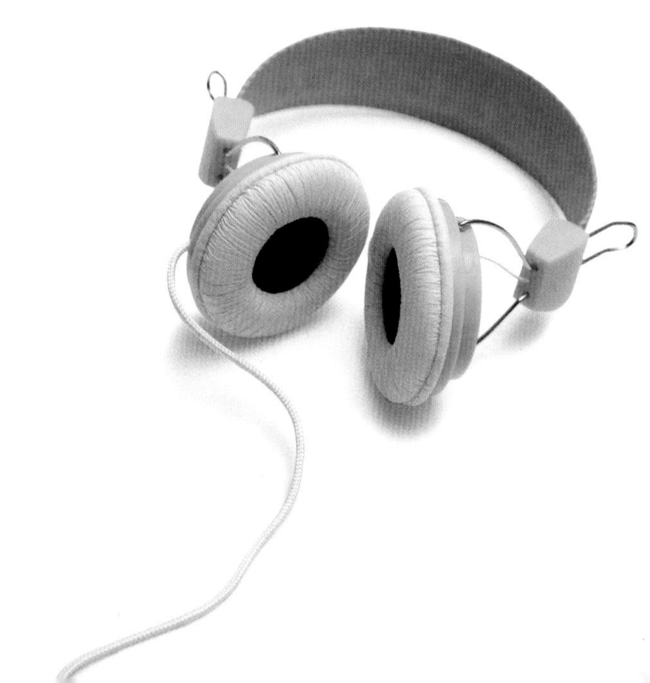

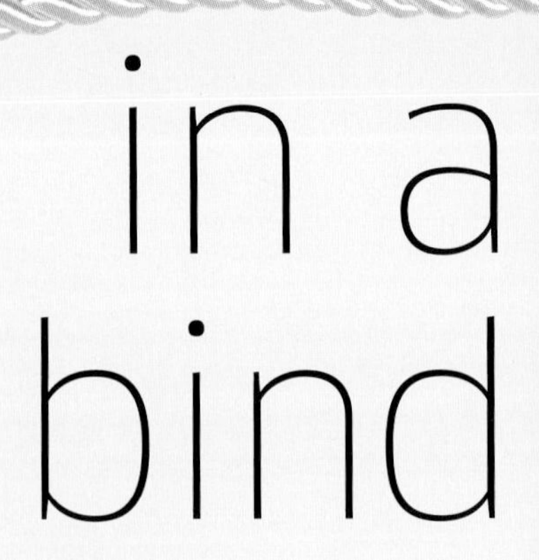

in a bind

We know you mean business when you come to bed with a pair of handcuffs. The thrill for us is that it takes dominance to the next level. If we're tied to the bed/chair/table, surrender really is our only option.

* Try **cuffing or tying him** wrist-to-wrist and ankle-to-ankle. Or tie him to the bedposts in the notorious **spread-eagle position**—you can access his best parts this way.

* **Tease him mercilessly** with **tongue flicks, kisses, bites, sucks, and strokes.** Or, if you could use some me-time, just **hop on top** and enjoy.

on tape

Hand him a roll of bondage tape and ask him to "dress" you. (Bondage tape is like sticky tape except it sticks only to itself so there is no pain involved!)

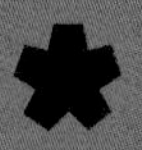

His job is to create the **tightest, kinkiest dress** by winding the tape around **your naked body.** Encourage him to leave gaps at certain strategic points so he can **kiss and touch** you. If you're fresh out of bondage tape, **try plastic wrap.**

Use your bondage tape to **tie his wrists** to the bed. Or behind his back. Then he is **completely at your mercy.**

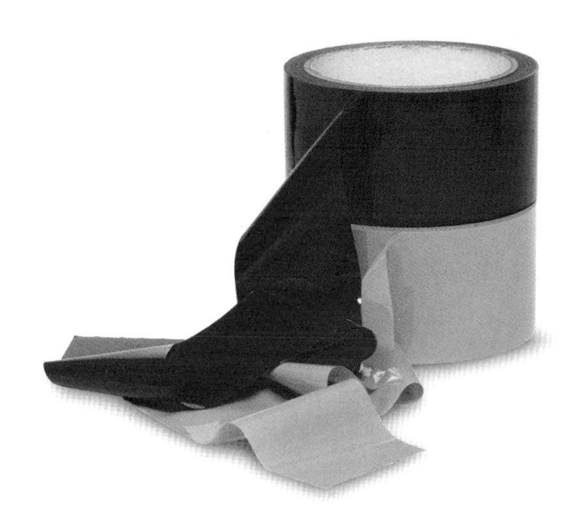

three ir

Threesomes: We make no apology, they're way up there on our list of hot fantasies. So if you want to make us crazy with pleasure, suggest some girl-on-boy-on-girl action.

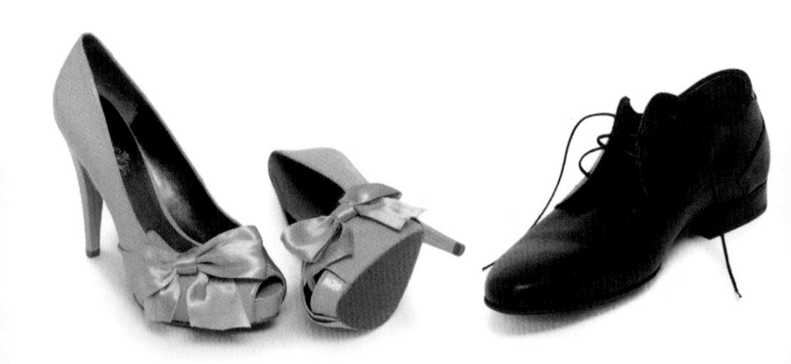

the bed

* **"It started** after a **party.** The **three of us** made out **for hours...**it was the most **memorable night of my life."**

* **"She and her friend** put a blindfold on me. After each **kiss, lick, or bite,** they asked, **'Guess who?'"**

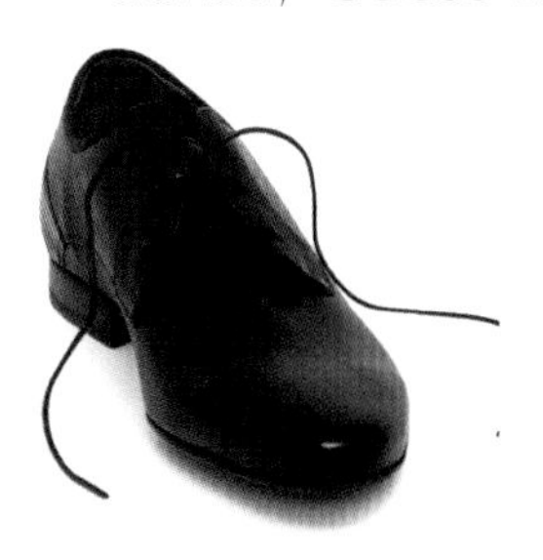

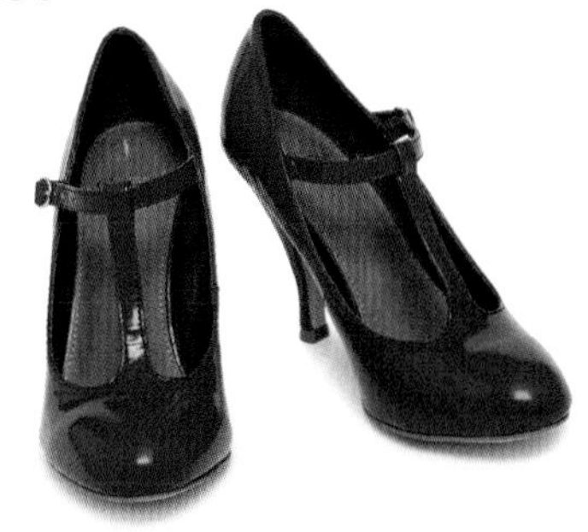

a touch of

Something about the look, smell, and feel of leather shouts “kinky” to us.

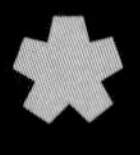

For beginner level kinkiness, wear a **leather belt.** He can **grab hold** of it **midaction.**

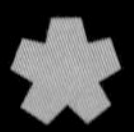

For **advanced raunch,** come to bed in a **leather corset** or **dog collar.**

leather

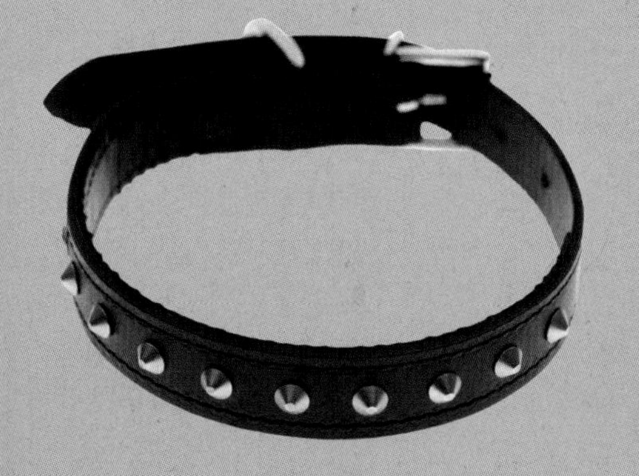

the first rule of S&M

don't

Before you throw yourself into some **bondage, spanking, or S&M,** agree on a "safe" word beforehand. Choose something silly, like **"lollipop."** Something sensible like **"stop"** might not work because you might want to shout that as **part of the kinky fun...**

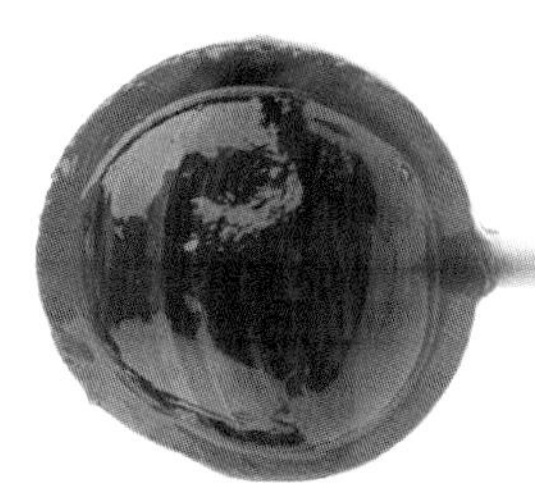

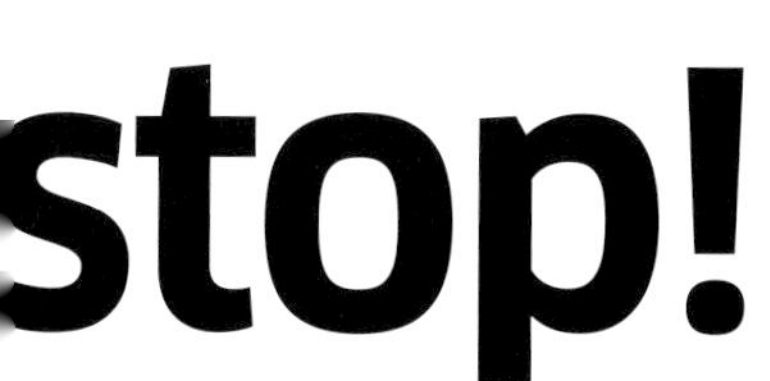
stop!

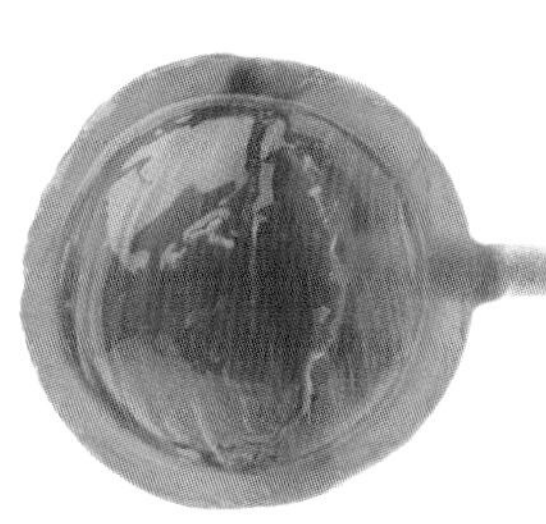

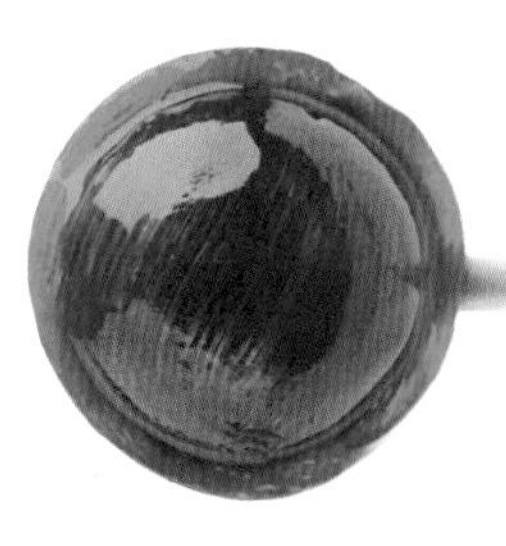

slavish devotion

Make him smile by offering to be his sex slave for the night. Tell him he can ask for whatever he wants (within reason). We will return the favor.

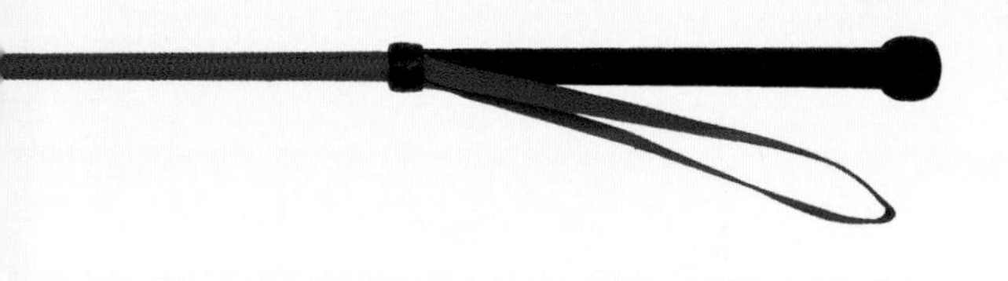

Get **dressed up** for the occasion. Try **wearing** a Venetian-style **masquerade mask**. It looks **gorgeously exotic** and **alluring,** and helps you both get into the **role-play.**

If **total submission** works for both of you, start on all fours and **crawl seductively** in his direction. Address him as **"master"** and **see what happens...**

going

Going to be apart for a while? Send him off with a sexy video of the two of you for him to discover in his suitcase.

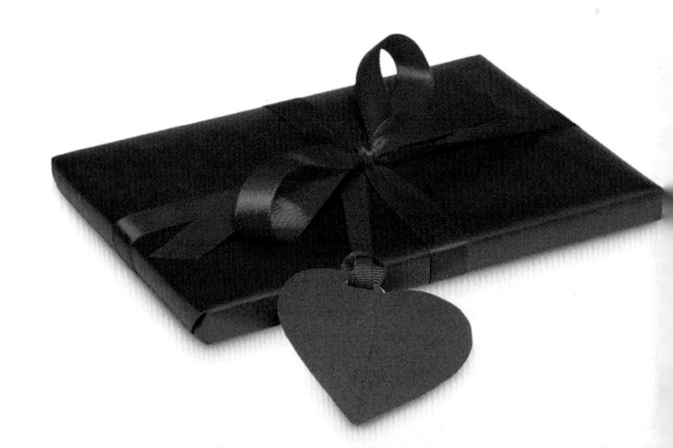

away gift

Make your film without him knowing. Film the two of you in a stunning sequence of **positions and moves.** It'll make for explosive viewing later.

Or try the old-school option: Tuck a **sexy photograph** into his bag for a **bedtime surprise.**

party night

You don't have to be into group sex and swinging to throw a sex party. You just need the two of you, a locked bedroom door, a supply of sexy goodies, and a naughty attitude.

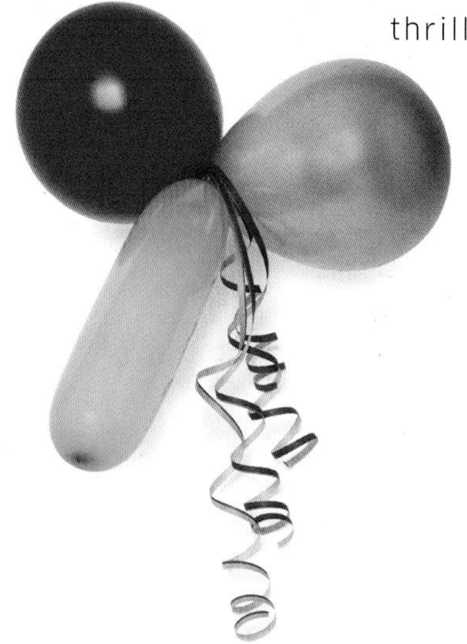

“One night a month we go over the top: **sex toys, videos, costumes, cocktails, and massage oil.”**

“Most of the time we’re **sweet and loving** in bed, but every now and then, **we agree that anything goes.”**

after

The next best thing to having **really great sex** is, in our opinion, thinking about the really great sex that we've had. In fact, sometimes **it's all we think about**. A good sex memory will last us until we're old and gray. Or at least until we make the next one.

glow

I once had incredible web cam sex. My girlfriend **video-called me and stripped.** When she was nearly naked her best friend came in and kissed her. Gorgeous!

My girlfriend surprised me with a **quickie just before we went** out. I grinned for the rest of the night.

I told my girlfriend I'd always fantasized about **sex on the beach.** So she indulged me by throwing a pop-up tent onto the sand and **pulling me inside.** She pushed me on my back, said "sshhh," and just climbed on top.

The **naughtiest** present I ever got was a Japanese sex chair. Instead of a seat it had wide elastic bands so that my girlfriend could sit on top while I penetrated her from below. **Weightless sex is sublime.**

My girlfriend knows I've got a fetish for girls in kinky nurse uniforms. So she threw a surprise party with a nurse/doctor dress code. **I was in heaven.**

My girlfriend once asked me to make an erotic film of her while **staying fully dressed** and concentrating on the camera work. She gave the **sexiest performance I've ever seen.** Then we had amazingly fast sex on the carpet!

My girlfriend and I went to see a **sex show** on vacation. We both agreed it was really seedy. Then we went back to our hotel room and **had the most fantastic sex**.

My girlfriend once booked a private sauna for us. She gave me the most **amazing naked massage.** Then, when we were both **drenched in sweat and oil**, she slipped onto my lap and rocked her way to orgasm.

My girlfriend played a very sexy trick on me. She **tied my hands and ankles together,** turned on an erotic video, and then left me by myself. Thankfully, she came back to **finish what she started**.

We were once having dinner at home. Out of the blue, my girlfriend **slipped out of her chair,** crawled underneath the table, and gave me a **surprise blow job** while I was eating.

picture credits

The publisher would like to thank the following for their kind permission to reproduce their photographs:

(Key: a-above; b-below/bottom; c-center; f-far; l-left; r-right; t-top)

1 Fotolia: Okea (br). 2 Getty Images: Rosemary Calvert (c). 5 Fotolia: Kramografie (br). 12-13 Corbis: Ocean. 16 Dreamstime.com: Kadrof (cl). 18-19 Corbis: Ocean. 21 Getty Images: Rosemary Calvert (bl). 23 Fotolia: FocalPoint (bc). 24 Corbis: Ocean (bl). 30 Getty Images: artpartner-images (br). 32 Corbis: Image Source (clb). 36-37 iStockphoto.com: EasyBuy4u. 41 Corbis: Glowimages (cb). 42 Corbis: Timothy Hogan (c). 46 Corbis: Jack Miskell Photography (c). 49 Corbis: Imagemore Co. (crb). 50 Fotolia: Anna Omelchenko (bl). 52 Fotolia: Vankad (bc). 54 Getty Images: Davies and Starr (cb). 56 Getty Images: Brand X Pictures (bc). 66 Fotolia: Michael Brown (clb). 68 Getty Images: moodboard (bl). 74 Getty Images: Burazin (c). 77 Fotolia: Elnur (tr). 84 Getty Images: Image Source (bc). 87 Getty Images: Stockbyte (br). 90-91 Getty Images: Ichiro. 93 Getty Images: Alex Cao (bc). 94 Getty Images: Tony Cordoza (cb). 97 Getty Images: Image Source (cb). 104 Corbis: Image source (br). 113 Corbis: Image source (br). 114 Getty Images: Caspar Benson (bl). 119 Getty Images: Annabelle Breakey (tr). 126 Corbis: Heide Benser (cl). 129 Fotolia: Rafa Irusta (c). 130 Getty Images: Rosemary Calvert (bl). 132 Getty Images: Thinkstock Images (c). 135 Fotolia: blueee (crb). 137 Corbis: I Love Images (cb). Getty Images: Grant Hamilton (bc). 139 Fotolia: andrej_sv (bc). 143 Alamy Images: Martin Lee (bc). 144 Fotolia: karandaev (bc). 146 Corbis: Ocean (bl). 149 Getty Images: Davies and Starr (c). 153 Fotolia: Skazka Grez (cb). 155 Getty Images: Maciej Toporowicz, NYC (bc). 160-161 Getty Images: Brian Hagiwara. 162 Getty Images: Jose Luis Pelaez (cb) 170 Fotolia: AndersonRise (bl). 176 Getty Images: Studio Box (bc). 179 Corbis: amanaimages (c). 184 Getty Images: Don Farrall (c). 190 Getty Images: Richard Boll (cb). 196-197 Alamy Images: jayfish. 202 Alamy Images: SDBprive (c). 211 Dreamstime.com: Ivonnewierink (ca). 212 Fotolia: Margrit Hirsch (c). 225 Corbis: Ocean (bc). 227 Getty Images: Robert Kirk (cb)

Jacket images: Front: Fotolia: lucielang c